Explorations in
Psychoneuroimmunology

SEMINARS IN PSYCHIATRY

Series Editor

Milton Greenblatt, M.D.

Chief of Psychiatry
Professor of Psychiatry, UCLA
Los Angeles County-Olive View Medical Center
Department of Health Sciences
Sylmar, California

Other Books in Series:

Explorations in Psychoneuroimmunology

Ruth Lloyd
Research Associate, Goodwin Institute for
Cancer Research, Plantation, Florida

Consulting Editor
George Freeman Solomon, M.D.

Consultant in Immunology
Martin E. Dorf, Ph.D.

Series Editor
Milton Greenblatt, M.D.

Grune & Stratton, Inc.
Harcourt Brace Jovanovich, Publishers
Orlando   New York   San Diego   London
San Francisco   Tokyo   Sydney   Toronto

Grune & Stratton, Inc.
Orlando, Florida 32887

Distributed in the United Kingdom by
Grune & Stratton, Ltd.
24/28 Oval Road, London NW 1

Library of Congress Catalog Number   86-083362
International Standard Book Number   0-8089-1854-0
Printed in the United States of America
87   88   89   90   10   9   8   7   6   5   4   3   2   1

Acknowledgments

The author is indebted to a number of individuals who have contributed in important ways to the making of this book. She wishes to express her gratitude, first of all, to Dr. George Freeman Solomon, Professor of Psychiatry, University of California, Los Angeles, Adjunct Professor of Psychiatry, University of California, San Francisco, who not only first broached the possibility of this enterprise, but has been a careful and concerned editor throughout its realization. Dr. Milton Greenblatt, Professor of Psychiatry, University of California, Los Angeles, Chief of Psychiatry, Veterans Administration Hospital, Sepulveda, and Editor for the Series of which this book is a part, has offered unfailing support. The author is indebted, as well, to Dr. Martin E. Dorf, Professor of Pathology, Harvard Medical School, for his critique of those parts of the book that deal specifically with the intricacies of immune phenomena.

From the time of her first venture into the field, the author has enjoyed the support of Dr. Joel Warren, Director of the Goodwin Institute for Cancer Research, Plantation, Florida, who has acted both as teacher and as astute critic of her writings. Dr. Bernard H. Fox, Professor in the Department of Psychiatry, Boston University School of Medicine, has made two decisive contributions to this book: first, in having selected the author's earlier review paper, "Mechanisms of Psychoneuroimmunological Response," for his and Dr. Benjamin H. Newberry's 1984 publication, *Impact of Psychoendocrine Systems on Cancer and Immunity*; second, in having graciously agreed to read—with his inimitable eye to logic and accuracy—earlier drafts of the present manuscript. The author also extends a special thanks to Mr. James Gorman, Department of Biology, Yale University, for his perceptive commentary.

Beginning in 1983, the author has profited from a lively and productive association with Steven E. Locke, M.D., Department of Psychiatry, The Beth Israel Hospital, Boston. The activities of the Behavioral Immunology Study Group, of which Dr. Locke is a founder, and for which the author served, for a time, as a Co-Chairman, have been a source of learning and inspiration.

A review of this scope could not have been undertaken without the expert assistance of Ms. Peg Hewitt, whose skilled information retrieval made it possible to address a wide range of topics with confidence, knowing that, in the end, all would be securely anchored to an accurate body of bibliographic reference. The author has also been privileged to collaborate with Ms. Nancy Newman, who prepared both the Subject and Author Indices, and with Ms. Deborah Osnowitz, who assisted in the preparation of the Glossary.

The author wishes to thank her children, her daughter, Lloyd Scott, and her sons, Philip W. Scott and David Malcolm Scott, for their forbearance and good humor towards what has been the author's semi-presence at the ordinary and pleasurable rituals of family life.

Finally, the author wishes to express her deep appreciation to her husband, Dr. Albert F. Ax, Editor, *International Journal of Psychophysiology,* for his able and impartial critiques of a manuscript so long in progress. Most of all, for his quiet confidence that in fact, one day, a book would come to be.

Contents

Preface

Psychoneuroimmunology is a contemporary science that has captured the imagination of investigators from specialized areas of science and medicine who have abandoned the specialist's stance. Theirs is an inclusory view of health and illness: one, therefore, that, by tradition, psychiatry shares. To draw relationships between immunity and the emotional life is not to depart, in any fundamental sense, from that tradition.

The writing of this book was undertaken at a time when a research area that had been gathering momentum over a period of two decades, seemed suddenly to burst with new energy. General reviews can, at best, highlight principal ideas and broadly outline the main directions of inquiry in a given field of study. In this case, where advances are taking place simultaneously—and at what seems a constantly accelerating pace—along many research fronts, it would be attempting the impossible to fully credit all the many investigators working in the field. Throughout the text, therefore, where space has not allowed for direct citation, the reader will find references to review papers devoted to areas of specialty.

Collaborations between scientists and clinicians that join idea and expertise in a dispassionate spirit can create an atmosphere of brilliance, particularly where these collaborations are seemingly unconstrained by either institutional or geographical boundaries. To this felicitous atmosphere, out of which psychoneuroimmunology has emerged, contemporary biology has imparted a brilliance of its own.

Editor's Preface

Mastery of the literature, felicity of expression, and the wisdom to integrate comprehensive knowledge in a complex growing field, typifies this prodigious work by Ruth Lloyd on Psychoneuroimmunology. This field was in its infancy when most of the doctors now practicing medicine matriculated. Today, it is a subject growing and changing so rapidly that no one can afford to neglect it. What was needed was a book written by a single author with unquestioned command of the literature who could also teach in a sophisticated, authoritative, and lucid style. When you read this volume, I think you will agree that Ruth Lloyd is a discovery of the first magnitude. Thus, we are understandably proud to present her major work under the imprimatur of the Grune & Stratton *Seminars in Psychiatry* series.

Milton Greenblatt, M.D.
Series Editor
Seminars in Psychiatry

September, 1986

Introduction

The idea that emotionally distressing episodes in the course of a human life can be associated with physical malaise, ill health, even with life-threatening illness, is an old idea. It is an integral part of a "folk wisdom" that presumes an interconnection between personal travail, loss of sanguineness, and decline in physical vigor. There is a general awareness, for example, that the experience of conjugal bereavement can increase the likelihood of morbidity and mortality in the bereaved, and that the recently widowed spouse is at increased risk of illness and early death. Given this understanding of a personal vulnerability that can touch both mind and body, it should not come as a source of astonishment that other severely stressful experiences of separation and loss may have similarly adverse *physiological* consequences.

This association between psychological trauma and compromised health status is now documented in an extensive clinical literature. Research questions formulated from the clinical observations amassed in this literature have provided the foundation for psychosomatic medicine. Do antecedents of disease reside in genetic constitution? Are there characteristics of personality specific to a given disease? Or, to place the question in the wider context, can discordance between the psychology of the individual and the pervading cultural ethos that inexorably shapes an individual life contribute to physical disease?

These questions are now being addressed with a new enthusiasm and exactness. Recent advances in our basic understanding of the immune system and in techniques of immune assessment, paralleled by important breakthroughs in genetics, cellular and molecular biology, neurophysiology, and neurochemistry, promise to *explain* the psychophysiological mechanisms underlying the psychosomatic concept. At the very least, the astonishing pace of discovery in these fundamental sciences may soon more fully explicate how idiosyncratic perception of "self," in relation to all that is contradistinctive from "self," can either protect or undermine physical well-being under conditions of life crisis. Most important, a theoretical foundation is being laid down to support the development of strategies for the treatment and prevention of stress-related disease.

As a consequence of this general ferment in the biological sciences (all biological research now benefiting from the techniques of biotechnology), the question of mind-body interaction in disease susceptibility has come under renewed scrutiny in clinical medicine and the behavioral sciences.

Investigators working in the evolving interdisciplines of psycho-neuroimmunology and neuroimmunomodulation recognize that the scope of recent information gained on characteristics of the immune response, particularly as this response relates to nervous and endocrine system function, has opened up a new perspective on the "mind-body problem" in general, and on the complexities of psychosomatic disease etiology in particular. This knowledge has also led to the realization that an entire complex of factors associated with personal crisis may affect immunity, such as prolonged emotional upset, changed habits of social interaction and personal care, an individual's relative success in coping with unaccustomed stress, etc.

It is now possible to evaluate immune competence, over time, with psychological evaluation, making possible the kind of comprehensive stress profile that should at last illuminate one of the more tantalizing puzzles in clinical medicine and stress research: namely, the extent to which individual differences in adaptation—differences shaped by personality, attitude, and behavior—predispose to illness, to wellness (Weiner, 1977). Moreover, as a result of newly available techniques for the assessment of immune status, immunological assay can now be carried out in *anticipation* of emotional upheaval, at the time of actual crisis, as well as during recovery from crisis.

In at least two respects, the application of these methods to the prospective evaluation of individuals at risk represents a most significant breakthrough. First of all, prognostic evaluative tools will enable health professionals of a psychosomatic persuasion to divest themselves of the "embarrassing infirmity of prediction" (Medawar, 1984, p. 4) that has acted as a constraint to their clinical effectiveness and confidence in the past. Secondly, with prognostic efficacy at its command, psychosomatic medicine acquires one of the indispensable and distinguishing characteristics of a true science. The future does indeed hold promise for the development of a comprehensive theory of disease that would be at once "functional, historical, and predictive" (Weiner, 1977, p. xii).

This book, in common with other contemporary writings on the subject, will posit a multifactoral concept of disease, *all* disease, taking into account the impact of immune system responsivity in much disease etiology. Here, one need only call to mind the many immunologically-resisted diseases, infectious and neoplastic, as well as diseases resulting from immunological aberration, such as the allergies and autoimmune disorders, to realize the breadth of the contemporary perspective.

It will be relevant to our general thesis to sketch out functional relationships among the three principal integrative systems of the body, nervous, endocrine, and immune. Structural, i.e., anatomic, connection between the brain and the primary and secondary tissues of immunity will be described, as will those chemical commonalities among the systems that imply commonalities of function.

It is impossible to view these common features and interconnections without seeing possible mechanisms for psychologically-induced changes in immune function. For example, it is a point of considerable interest that the neural and neuroendocrine substrates of those emotions and mood states likely to be associated with trauma, experienced loss, or failure of psychological defenses, also play a role in immune dysfunction.

But that the parts that make up the whole should be well understood, we will first outline the principal characteristics and activities of the immune system, describing its complex of organs (which is simple enough in its organization), as well as the roles played by its multifarious cell populations (which are not). How the immune system works, and how its operations affect, and are affected by, other physiological systems is basic knowledge that applies to the broader issue of mind-body interaction in the maintenance of health.

Solomon (1985) has formulated a number of hypotheses regarding the modulatory interaction of bodily systems. He has argued, for example, that if a functional relationship does indeed exist between the central nervous system and the immune system, hormones and other substances regulated or elaborated by the CNS should influence immune mechanisms. It should be possible, as a consequence, to show receptor sites for neurotransmitters and neuroendocrine hormones on the surface membranes of activated immune (immunocompetent) cells. What is more, hormones produced by the principal organ of the immune system, the thymus gland, should not only be influenced by central mediator substances, but should in turn influence the chemical equilibrium of central structures.

The premise that psychological state can affect immunity would gain further support were it found that the experimental manipulation of appropriate target areas of the central nervous system has immunologic consequences. By the same token, products of immune system activation should elicit reactive bioelectric phenomena within the brain.

As corollary to this latter observation, diseases of immunologic aberration should be accompanied, at times, by psychological and/or neurological symptoms. The converse should also prove to be true. Additionally, there should be a likelihood that biochemical and functional similarities exist between substances that modulate brain function and reactivity (the neuropeptides, for example), and substances having comparable biologic action within immune system components (hormone-like products of lymphocytes, for example). To these propositions one might add the implicit assumption that endocrine, neuroendocrine, and immune mechanisms of aging should exhibit degrees of congruence.

The capacity of the immune system to learn, to respond to stimulus contingencies, has been demonstrated in the behavioral conditioning of immune reactions in laboratory animals. In evaluating this finding, two principal contemporary investigators of the phenomenon believe that it demonstrates "an intimate and virtually unexplored relationship between the central nervous system and immunologic processes...a mechanism that may be involved in the complex pathogenesis of psychosomatic disease" (Ader & Cohen, 1975, pp. 338-339). A rationale for therapeutic intervention therefore presents itself, for despite the preliminary nature of clinically relevant data produced from this research thus far, therapeutic strategies are likely to be devised that would maintain, or restore, immune competence. Given the fact that the significant pairing in the conditioning paradigm (that is, the pairing of a neutral stimulus with an unconditioned response) should, at least in principle, operate in both immune suppression and immune enhancement, and granting our position that mental and physical function are ineluctably linked, it would certainly seem worthwhile to consider the possibility that these same principles of learning might be successfully applied in the psychotherapeutic setting.

From a more general standpoint, it should now be possible to more readily conceptualize fluctuations in immune function in relation to behavioral change, to view each as taking place within a social milieu, each as being continuously influenced by the symbolic climate of everyday life. Or—to express the same point in more technical language—to concede that the two processes, immune system activity and behavior, are in varying degree, susceptible to learning within a stimulus context.

Finally, it should prove fruitful to incorporate the deep knowledge of human personality that is a hallmark of psychodynamic psychiatry and psychology into the rather complicated conceptual framework presently being shaped by psychoneuroimmunological research. To this end, and to the extent to which such incorporation is presently justifiable, it will be the task of the author to substantiate the notion that attributes of personality may act in concert with exogenous, experiential factors to influence immune competency, and that individual styles of coping with adversity may have immunologic consequences.

REFERENCES

Ader, R., & Cohen, N. Behaviorally conditioned immunosuppression. *Psychosomatic Medicine,* 1975, 37 (4), 333-340.

Medawar, P. B. *The Limits of Science.* New York: Harper & Row, Publishers, 1984.

Solomon, G. F. The emerging field of psychoneuroimmunology—With a special note on AIDS. *Advances,* 1985, 2 (1), 6-19.

Weiner, H. *Psychobiology and Human Disease.* New York: Elsevier, 1977.

Chapter 1

Historical Perspective: Notes on the Development of an Interdiscipline

Psychoneuroimmunology is a newly differentiated field in modern medical science devoted to the exploration of ancient truths. The idea that reason and emotion, the primary emergent properties of the brain, might affect immunity has infused the philosophy and practice of healing for millenia. The Ayurveda of ancient India, for example, is based on the twin notions that wellness reflects a balance of life forces, a unity of Man and Universe, and that illness, by contrast, reflects a disequilibrium, or, at worst, a disharmony, of these same forces. In this "science of life," restraint of the mind from harmful pursuits is a central therapeutic principle that applies as much to the preservation of health as to the healing of bodily ills (Caraka, 7th century, B.C.E.; Shukla, Solomon, & Doshi, l979).

The development of psychoneuroimmunology is more directly indebted, however, to closely related concepts of the more recent past, specifically to those that have formed the framework of psychosomatic theory over the past 50 years (Murray, 1977). By placing emphasis on the psychologic and sociocultural *antecedents* to disease—in other words, by documenting the effects of such disparate variables as characteristics of personality, perception of self, genetic predisposition, specific organ susceptibility, and total life experience (Weiner, 1977)—this branch of clinical medicine has reaffirmed, in principle, the beliefs of the ancient seers.

Open to criticism as reversionary, this earnest attempt at synthesis has nonetheless had a salutary effect, for it has helped to counteract the mechanistic, emphatically physiopathologic orientation of nineteenth cen-

1

tury medicine (Alexander, 1939). Unfortunately, the undoubted strengths to be found in this perspective on disease etiology are also its weakness: where it has had descriptive value, it has lacked predictive power (Weiner, 1977).

Whereas psychosomatic medicine might rightly be called its philosophic home, psychoneuroimmunology has deliberately broadened its theoretical base by incorporating precepts from physiological psychology on stress and disease in laboratory animals. It is thus the beneficiary of a wealth of data, obtained through the concurrent measurement of emotionality, overt behavior, and one or another physiologic parameter, on integral response patterns observed in relation to a variety of stressors recorded over time (see Monjan, 1981; Riley, Fitzmaurice, & Spackman, 1981; Solomon & Amkraut, 1981, for recent reviews).

Insights on the relationship between psychologic and *immunologic* profiles in immunologically-mediated diseases in humans were a first important contribution to the new science. In a landmark group of studies carried out in the 1960s, Solomon and Moos, two pioneers in "psychoimmunology"—as they then dared to call it—astutely associated new findings in endocrinology and immunology with a research literature on psychologic assessment of persons afflicted with the systemic autoimmune disorder, rheumatoid arthritis (Moos, 1964).

A number of consonant observations guided these early investigations. One: healthy siblings of rheumatoid arthritis patients demonstrated both robust emotional health *and* the presence of rheumatoid factor (anti-immunoglobulin), a finding that implied that manifest disease must reflect the combined effect of emotional decompensation (failure of defense mechanisms) and immunologic predisposition (Moos & Solomon, 1965a, 1965b; Solomon & Moos, 1964, 1965). Two: emotional distress and fragile ego defense structure observed in arthritic patients were characteristics not unlike those found in patients with other disorders of immunity. Psychologic features of this type had been noted in patients with ulcerative colitis (Engel, 1955), Graves' disease (Mandelbrote & Wittkower, 1955), systemic lupus erythematosus (SLE) (McClary, Meyer, & Weitzman, 1955), and the hemorrhagic (purpuric) condition, autoerythrocyte sensitization, this last having been described as a "psychosomatic entity" (Agle & Ratnoff, 1962). Three: psychological profiles of the arthritic patient group under study, and of patients with cancer (Leshan & Worthington, 1956), showed close similarity. Four: depression and emotional upset in response to "naturally occurring" psychological stressors had been found to be associated with elevated adrenal cortical steroid hormone levels in humans (Hamburg, 1962). Five: animal research had shown an apparently clear-cut relationship between elevated cortisol levels and compromised immune function (Hirschhorn et al., 1963; Vessey, 1964)—a relationship, by the way, that has subsequently been found to be less than clear-cut (Monjan, 1981). And finally, preliminary work, later to be more fully substantiated (Fudenberg, 1968), had suggested that autoimmunity was associated with diminished immunologic competence (Dixon, Feldman, & Vasquez, 1959, 1961).

AUTOIMMUNE DISEASE AS HEURISTIC MODEL

Through the felicitous juxtaposition of hypothesis and fact, Solomon and Moos succeeded, in a sense, in touching the lodestone: that is to say, they first perceived, then documented, *how* psychogenic stress might alter the internal state of the organism to such a degree that normal immunologic homeostasis (in this case, immune tolerance to autologous, or "self," antigens) could either be compromised or altogether undermined (Solomon, 1981b). It appeared that individual coping style and a constellation of personality attributes might correlate with a more or less stable, idiosyncratic immunologic profile. The ramifications leading from this conclusion were many, but, at the very least, it seemed likely that new insights were now to be gained on the nature of the "transducer chain" of events (Delbrück, cited in Bergman et al., 1969) connecting conscious experience to endocrine, neurochemical, and immunologic process.

If there were a weak link in the chain, it would reside in the validity and reliability of psychologic measurement, and in methodologic problems involved in the assessment of state and trait in human subjects. These difficulties were not thought insurmountable, however, and it was hoped that future research in the area might incorporate some of the features that had given these first studies their breadth and strong interdisciplinary emphasis (Moos & Solomon, 1965a).

In fact, it cannot have escaped notice that these interesting and potentially important observations were made (and published) 20 years before psychoneuroimmunology became an established, active field of research. The particular amalgam of knowledge and influence through which an area of science succeeds in being introduced, then promoted, is a topic beyond the scope and purpose of this book. Suffice it to say that another full decade was to pass before speculations with respect to the autoimmune phenomenon itself—a phenomenon directly antithetical to Paul Erlich's notion of "horror autotoxicus" (Erlich, 1900)—were to be placed on a firm foundation of experimental evidence; let alone speculations on psychoimmunologic phenomena!

In time, the production of tissue-damaging autoantibodies in autoimmune disease came to be understood as a failure in inhibitory feedback in the lymphocyte network, discriminatory disturbance within that network (Langman, 1984), and excessive proliferation of a single immune cell type (Talal, 1977, 1978). Some, but by no means all, of the deviations from normal immunologic control in diseases of this type were found to include a decrease in T "suppressor," relative to T "helper," cell function, B cell hyperresponsivity, increased numbers of immunoglobulin-secreting cells, and production of autoantibodies much above clinically normal levels (Rosenberg, Steinberg, & Santoro, 1984; Talal, 1980; Theofilopoulos, 1984).

The question of autoimmune disease etiology remains a challenge to this day. Among other concerns, the immunologist has the task of fully understanding the changing mechanisms of self-tolerance during fetal, neonatal, and adult life (Malkovsky & Medawar, 1984). The psychoneuroimmunologist, on the other hand, must focus his or her attention on reactive patterns of emotion and behavior that may predispose an individual to autoimmunity. To quote from a 1984 article on the topic:

> When one considers the myriad chemical classes of self antigens, the variations in plasma concentration of these antigens, the ontogenetic appearance (and disappearance) of these markers, and the heterogeneity of B...and T cells which must "learn" to see these antigens as self, it is apparent that multiple pathways must exist to insure the integrity of the host (Scott, 1984, p. 69).

Another important contribution to psychoneuroimmunology has come from the research specialty of neuroimmunomodulation (Spector, 1980). Here, the techniques of neurophysiology and immunophysiology have been combined to extend our knowledge of immune system connection to other physiologic systems; most importantly, its connection to and from loci within the central nervous system governing motivation, emotion, and mood. The first bold experiments in this field were pioneered in the Soviet Union by Korneva and Khai in the 1960s with the express purpose of showing "the organization and regulation of immunologic processes within the whole organism" (Spector & Korneva, 1981, pp. 452-453).

Finally, there exists today a sizable literature describing the direct effect imposed on immune system function by what appears to be a continually expanding repertoire of physiochemical mediators of the "stress response," substances such as neurotransmitters, neuropeptides, histamine, steroids, prostaglandins, etc. Every effort is being made to understand the indirect effects of these substances on "second messenger" systems within body cells, including lymphocytes. Perhaps the most difficult challenge of all has been to identify the countless choice points and end-sequences through which immunocompetent cells recognize self components as either "toleragens" (to which they need not respond), or "immunogens" (to which they must appropriately respond).

A DEBT TO IMMUNOLOGY

As an interdiscipline, psychoneuroimmunology represents a significant departure from previous attempts at synthesis in the biological and behavioral sciences. It has allowed a fresh examination of the perturbations in psychoendocrine regulation that jeopardize immunologic protection of the physiologic "self." Also, to state the converse, its enlargement of the psychosomatic concept has stimulated basic research on stress-related derangements in intercellular communication that, by either impeding or subverting recognition of pathogen and/or mutagen, threaten the stability of other complementary homeostatic controls.

Today, psychoneuroimmunologic research has attained a high level of sophistication and a breadth of outlook that augurs well for the future success of the new field. Already, the list of participants in the multidiscipline is long: psychiatry, psychology, neuropsychology, neurophysiology, neuroendocrinology, functional anatomy, cellular and molecular immunology, immunopharmacology, biophysics, microbiology, chronobiology, psychooncology, endocrinology, embryology, biochemistry, immunogenetics—to name a few. Needless to say, a single research program, as organized by a multidisciplinary team of scientists, is ably equipped to erect multiple parameters (e.g., behavioral, neuroendocrine, and immune) for simultaneous observation and analysis. Not surprisingly, "hard" data to support the underlying premises of the fledgling science are accummulating at a rapid pace.

The science of immunology has provided the spark to this lively state of affairs. There can be little doubt that, excepting its new energy and increased sophistication in its research tools (Rabkin & Struening, 1976), psychoneuroimmunology is the direct beneficiary of remarkable advances in immunology, paralleled by like advances in genetics. For this reason, a brief overview of historical highlights in immunology should provide an appropriate perspective from which to evaluate the growth of the younger science. Furthermore, as we shall see, the histories of the two sciences are intertwined.

PRELUDE TO THE GREAT SCHISM

The history of immunology, as an independent discipline, makes plain that, during the fifty-odd years spanning its beginnings, the basic premises of the science were defined, heuristic paths of investigation were laid down, and theories concerning immunologic function were formulated to a degree sufficient to generate vigorous scientific debate along lines of argument pursued to this day. These were years that spanned the lifetimes of estimable pioneers in modern bacteriology (the basic science to modern immunology), years that saw the formation of great research institutions in England and on the Continent.

Given our hard won contemporary view that physiologic systems make up a complex, an interdependent whole (Besedovsky & Sorkin, 1977; Lloyd, 1984a, 1984b), the early days of immune studies were days of vision, vision later lost. For, in truth, psychoneuroimmunology existed as a nascent interdiscipline in the 1920s, this circumstance having come to pass quite simply from the fact that physiologists saw the immune system as being susceptible to governance by the brain—hence, in no way unique among body systems.

For example, in experiments carried out in 1926 at the Pasteur Institute in Paris, Metal'nikov and Chorine succeeded in applying the principles and procedures of Pavlovian conditioning to the *simultaneous* elicitation of both immunologic and nonspecific, physiologic defense reactions in laboratory animals.[*] To quote from the authors' forthright premise: "the basis of immunity is formed by defensive reactions of the various cells of the organism" (Metal'nikov & Chorine, 1926, p. 263).

The point of interest here is that Metal'nikov's conviction that the complexity of immunologic response made "l'intervention du système nerveux" an essential requisite to their regulation (Metal'nikov, 1934) was not brought into serious question at the time of his and Chorine's initial experiments; nor was the theoretical basis of subsequent research undertaken to expand upon and replicate their original findings (see Ader, 1981, for a comprehensive review of corroborative evidence). Rather, it was largely with respect to the unanswered question of *mechanism* or mechanisms underlying the observed phenomena that this provocative research lay open to criticism, some of it severe (for an account of this controversy, see Ader, 1981).

---

[*]In faithful adherence to the methods originated in "the remarkable works of J. Pavlov and his students," Metal'nikov and Chorine introduced an innocuous, external (conditioned) stimulus in repeated temporal association with an involuntary immune response (conditioned reflex) to administered antigen (i.e., tapioca, B-anthracoids, or staphylococcus filtrate), the conditioned stimulus being rendered capable, in time, of eliciting a like reflex in the absence of antigen. Immune reactivity was measured by leukocyte count of exudate of the peritoneum, the site of antigen injection.

Modern scientific dogma was, after all, already well in place: "It is characteristic of science to reduce incessantly the number of unexplained phenomena." So Louis Pasteur himself had stated 45 years previous as introductory comment to his extensive reports on the fermentation of yeast (Pasteur, 1879). Dogma is formidable in its influence. As far as the classical conditioning (i.e., higher cortical mediation) of immunologic response was concerned, the case remained fixed in controversy for a number of years (Dolin et al., 1960). Only recently has the subject been reexplored in experiments on aversively conditioned immunosuppression by Robert Ader and his colleagues (Ader & Cohen, 1981, 1985)—research undertaken, one might hope, in a somewhat less disputatious atmosphere.

Hence, a kind of contretemps (quite literally) positioned Metal'nikov's work and intellectual stance, as well as that of his collaborators and colleagues, in what might be termed a "time-lock." The pity here was that the evidence of mechanism linking immune function and psychologic process—for want of which modern psychosomatic research suffered a similar, if briefer, eclipse—became encapsulated.

This interlude in the story of psychoneuroimmunology provides an excellent example of the periodicity of ideas that characterizes scientific pursuit no less than other equally rarified realms of human endeavor. The rather disjointed development of psychoneuroimmunology as a distinct research discipline reflects the seemingly cyclic episodes of consolidation (and their opposite) that occur between differing areas of investigation, such episodes often reflecting prevailing attitudes within the scientific community at large.

IMMUNOLOGY AS A WORLD APART

The concept of immunologic response as part of a general systems interaction was obscured in the years that followed. In truth, immunology came to be viewed as "an island of science almost entire of itself" (Haurowitz, 1980, p. 15), and the immune system as an autonomous system, independent of the brain.

Antecedent to, and during the period in which the behavioral (Pavlovian) approach to immunologic phenomena languished in controversy, the study of immunity was beginning to expand beyond its beginnings in bacteriology. In place of an emphasis on taxonomy and the search for the "morbid agents" responsible for such dread diseases as cholera (Louis Pasteur, 1867), typhoid (Georges F. I. Widal & Arthur Sicar, 1896), and tuberculosis (Jean-Antoine Villemin, 1868), attention turned to possible mechanisms whereby immunity itself might be explained, this reorientation resulting from a series of fortuitous discoveries, one of the earliest of which had occurred nearly 70 years before (see Bellanti & Kadlec, 1985; Graber, 1984; Silverstein, 1979, for general historical background).

As is well known, the English surgeon, Edward Jenner, was renowned for his careful (and controversial) experimentation with the vaccination of cowpox (vaccinia) and smallpox (variola) viruses, having conducted "as strict an inquiry into the causes and effects of this singular malady as local circumstances would admit" (letter, published in Jenner, 1798). Jenner observed that "what renders the cowpox virus so extremely singular is that the person who has been thus affected is forever after secure from the infection of the smallpox; neither exposure to variolous effluvia, nor the insertion of the matter into the skin, producing this distemper." Within a decade of Jenner's initial discoveries, a first compulsory program of vaccination was introduced against the age-old scourge. It should be stressed that Jenner's researches resulted in a fastidiously detailed documention of the phenomenon of immunologic memory.

For the fledging science of immunology, one of the first true hallmarks of maturity occurred nearly a century after the publication of Jenner's work. In 1883, the Russian zoologist, Elie I.I. Metchnikoff, developed a *theory of cellular immunity* from a single, informed observation: namely, that foreign matter (in this case, a rose thorn thrust into the flesh of star fish larvae and *daphnia* crustacea) became subject to complete engulfment and digestion by motile cells, cells later identified as polymorphonuclear leukocytes and macrophages.

Shortly thereafter, a *theory of humoral immunity* grew out of the discovery by Emil A. von Behring and Shibasaburo Kitasato that the sera of animals immunized against diphtheria and tetanus exerted neutralizing, antitoxic effects. Theory and practice were then felicitously combined in the first large scale production of antisera in the aforementioned institutes, the Pasteur Institute (Paris), the Lister Institute (London), and, preeminently, the Behring Institute (Marburg, Germany), this last named after the Nobel Laureate,[*] von Behring, cofounder, with Kitasato, of serotherapy.

At this same time, Paul Erlich contributed his *side-chain theory* of immunity to explain antigen recognition by immune cells, believing it to be *chemically* mediated. Here lay the theoretical basis for the concept of antibody formation. Erlich was responsible, as well, for introducing the revolutionary idea that the surface membranes of macromolecules and body cells harbored active recognition components.

---

[*]Other early Nobel Laureates in immunology were Paul Ehrlich and Elie I.I. Metchnikoff (1908), Charles Robert Richet (1913), Jules J. B. V. Bordet (1919), and Karl Landsteiner (1930).

Within this same 20 year period, adverse, within-species, reaction to blood transfusion (red blood cell agglutination) came under intensive study by L. Landois and Jules J. B. V. Bordet. These investigators realized that the agglutination reaction illustrated the antigenic specificity of a particular cell type among individual members of the same species. They saw, too, that it provided still further evidence for a humoral mechanism in immunity.

In 1902, Karl Landsteiner succeeded in isolating the blood groups, A, B, O, and Rh factor, an outcome of his studies on blood type incompatibility among individual members of a species. Landsteiner also became a pioneer of immunochemistry, initiating a comprehensive series of experiments on the specificity and *immunogenicity* of artificial chemical groupings, or "conjugated antigens," recording their stimulation of antibody production in serologic reactions.

Simultaneous to Landsteiner's identification of blood types, Charles R. Richet and Paul J. Portier made the "absolutely unexpected" discovery that reexposure to an allergen (in this case, a glycerin extract of the tentacles of the sea anemone, *Actinaria*, injected in dogs) could inititate a rapid systemic, usually fatal, allergic ("anaphylactic") response, one that typically culminated in respiratory obstruction and profound vascular collapse. This one experiment forever altered the commonly held view that immunologic reactions to invasive antigen were universally defensive and protective to the host (Grabar, 1984; see also Bellanti & Kadlec, 1985; Silverstein, 1979, for historical background).

THE PENDULUM SWINGS

In time, bacteriology became a part of microbiology, and as one of many separate disciplines in the biological sciences, the science of immunology drew momentum and expertise from advances in other fields; most notably from biochemistry, cytology, virology, embryology, and genetics. As the years have passed, advances in immunology itself have proven to be sustained and dramatic.

Unfortunately, the consequences of this technological surge to the "nascent discipline" were not happy. In 1955, the Russian immunologist, G. V. Vygodchikov, "bemoaned the reductionistic approach that failed to consider the total organism within which immunologic processes were taking place" (Ader, 1981, p. 336-337). And are we, 30 years later, any broader in our point of view, despite the breadth of scientific knowledge we enjoy? To quote from a 1984 statement on the question by an eminent immunologist, a statement delivered as part of a critique on a 1984 collection of research and theoretical papers describing the impact of psycho-endocrine systems on immunity: "most immunologists are sensibly engaged in exploring the immune system itself...Only a few are interested in links between psyche and soma as far as immunology is concerned. For most immunologists, [the topic] will provide little which will affect their work or concepts" (Sorkin, 1984, p. 227).

The statement is itself extraordinary, given the evidence at hand. Nevertheless, in defense of this persistent insularity in science, it should be pointed out that there are enormous practical and methodological impediments to interdisciplinary research. Inevitably, such impediments have not only tended to discourage broad-based research undertakings of the latter kind, but have also undoubtedly inhibited the breadth of scientific outlook that would act as an generative force to such research.

At the same time, it cannot be overlooked that immunology has come to enjoy an enviable position in contemporary biological science, a position from which the ready exchange of ideas would seem all the more likely to take place. It is obvious, for example, that certain basic discoveries in immunology, as well as some of its more esoteric research techniques, have been ingeniously adapted to the research needs of other disciplines, with good result. As a case in point, the advent of cell fusion, i.e., the hybridization of antibody-producing cells and tumor (*myeloma*) cells (Köhler & Milstein, 1975, 1976), has had an impact on the biological sciences in general, and medical research in particular, that can only be described as spectacular. No less important is the contribution by immunology to the widespread use of radioimmunoassay, immunodiffusion, immunofluorescence, and immunoelectrophoresis in both basic and clinical research and diagnosis. As Felix Haurowitz (1980) has nicely expressed it: "immunology in this way has liquidated its debt to the basic sciences which provided it with these quantitative methods" (p. 14).

Perhaps inevitably, cross-fertilization between the sciences has so far been largely an exchange of techniques, minimumly one of ideas. Thus, there has been a ready acceptance of immunohistochemical technology, but what of the concepts guiding the research for which this technology was developed in the first place?

The mechanisms of psychoneuroimmunologic response offer an investigative challenge of quite considerable scope, wide and deep enough, perhaps, to overcome at least a few of the still-prevailing intellectual barriers in biomedical research. It may be that we shall at last be able, in the words of the immunologist, Alistair J. Cunningham (1983), to "test the explanatory power of our conventional reductionist techniques and try to devise new approaches where reductionism has failed" (p. 610).

Immunologic response appears to have been a silent partner in the psychoneuroendocrine reaction patterns that have been documented in countless multidisciplinary studies in psychobiology. It is time that studies on the interplay of psyche and soma should necessarily and routinely include the monitoring of immunologic function.

CONCLUSIONS

Immunology has profited from interaction with allied sciences that have advanced at pace more or less parallel to its own. Research on the stereochemistry of cell surface receptors, as well as impressive advances in protein and nucleic acid chemistry, are revealing the mechanisms of cell activation, growth, and differentiation in the various cell systems of the body, including the progenitor and effector cells of immunity. Each such cell system, it might be added, representing an independent scientific discipline!

Cell communication is the paramount question around which all other questions turn. How are control signals within and between cells to be defined? If communication takes place at the molecular level, as is assumed, what are the control molecules? What is the nature of receptor sites occupied by these molecules? And under what conditions are receptor structures present and viable?

With the knowledge that at least some of the mysteries of normal and abnormal cell communication are being unraveled, a sense of excitement prevails (Burgess, 1984). There is confidence, too, that technical problems involved in the chemical characterization, purification, and cloning of target cell or molecule for purposes of study and therapeutic application are surmountable problems, soon to be entirely solved.

Unquestionably, discoveries taking place at this research frontier will help to explain the impact of psychoendocrine factors on immunity. Likewise, stress-related disorders of autoimmunity should provide a rallying point for broadly conceived investigations in this area. If autoantigens (self-markers) and self-reactive effector lymphocytes are present under normal conditions (as, in truth, they are) (Cooke, Lydyard, & Roitt, 1983), what derangements of control systems (cellular, molecular, or both) are likely to trigger lymphocyte autoreactivity? It has been shown with respect to at least one lymphocyte subset (the B cells) that self-tolerance can "be broken with relative ease" (Cooke et al., 1983, p. 171). What triggers the break?

The chemical substrate of experienced stress may contribute to these derangements. It is not inconceivable that the surge of steroid hormones and neural humors characteristic of "adaptation syndromes" (Selye, 1946) is sufficient to bring about alterations in lymphocyte membrane receptor conformation.

There are powerful internal forces driven by emotion and perceptual set that undoubtedly play a crucial role in normal and pathologic process—control forces *external* to the minutae that have so long riveted the attention of scientists in basic medical research, immunology included. If we were to recall that conditioning, an event mediated by the psyche, can be both physiologically arousing *and* immunostimulatory, we might realize that the so-called rift between the "hard" and "soft" sciences is, in reality, no rift at all.

REFERENCES

Ader, R. An historical account of conditioned immunologic responses. In R. Ader (Ed.), *Psychoneuroimmunology*. New York: Academic Press, 1981, 321-352.

Ader, R., & Cohen, N. Conditioned immunopharmacological responses. In R. Ader (Ed.), *Psychoneuroimmunology*. New York: Academic Press, 1981, 281-319.

Ader, R., & Cohen, N. CNS-immune system interactions: Conditioning phenomena. *Behavior and Brain Sciences,* 1985, 8 (3), 379-395.

Agle, D. P., & Ratnoff, O. D. Purpura as psychosomatic entity. *Archives of Internal Medicine,* 1962, 109 (6), 685-694.

Alexander, F. Psychological aspects of medicine. *Psychosomatic Medicine,* 1939, 1 (1), 7-18.

Bellanti, J. A., & Kadlec, J. V. Introduction to immunology. In J. A. Bellanti (Ed.), *Immunology III*. Philadelphia: W. B. Saunders, 1985, 1-15.

Bergman, K., Burke, P. V., Cerda-Olmedo, E., David, C. N., Delbrück, M., Foster, K. W., Goodell, E. W., Heisenberg, M., Meissner, G., Zalokar, M., Dennison, D. S., & Shropshire, W. Phycomyces. *Bacteriology Review,* 1969, 33 (1), 99-157.

Besedovsky, H., & Sorkin, E. Network of immuneneuroendocrine interactions. *Clinical and Experimental Immunology,* 1977, 27 (1), 1-12.

Burgess, A. W. The complex mediators of cell growth and differentiation. *Immunology Today,* 1984, 5 (6), 155-158.

Caraka. *Caraka Sămhita*, 7th century, B.C.E. (Wisdom as expounded by Caraka, Physician-Seer. English translation from the Sanskrit by P. V. Sharma.) 1st edition. Varanasi, India: Chankhanbha Orientalia, 1981.

Cooke, A., Lydyard, P. M., & Roitt, I. M. Mechanisms of autoimmunity: A role for cross-reactive idiotypes. *Immunology Today,* 1983, 4 (6), 170-175.

Cunningham, A. J. Mind, body, and immune response. In R. Ader (Ed.), *Psychoneuroimmunology.* New York: Academic Press, 1981, 609-617.

Dixon, F. J., Feldman, J., & Vasquez, J. Immunology and pathogenesis of experimental serum sickness. *Cellular and Humoral Aspects of Hypersensitive States.* New York: Harper & Row, Publishers, 1959.

Dolin, A. O., Krylov, B. N., Luk'ianenko, V. I., & Flerov, B. A. New experimental data on the conditioned reflex reproduction and suppression of immune and allergic reactions. *Zhurnal Vysshei Nervnoi Deiatelno sti imeni I. P. Pavlova,* 1960, 10, 832-841. (in Russian)

Ehrlich, P. Croonian Lecture. On immunity with special reference to cell life. *Proceedings of the Royal Society (London),* 1900, LXVI (432), 424-448.

Engel, G. Studies of ulcerative colitis. III. Nature of the psychologic process. *American Journal of Medicine,* 1955, 19 (2), 231-256.

Fudenberg, H. H. Are autoimmune disorders immunologic deficiency states? *Hospital Practice,* 1968, 3 (1), 43-53.

Grabar, P. The historical background of immunology. In D. P. Stites, J. D. Stobo, H. H. Fudenberg, & J. V. Wells (Eds.), *Basic & Clinical Immunology.* 5th edition. Los Altos, California: Lange Medical Publications, 1984, 1-12.

Hamburg, D. A. Plasma and urinary corticosteroid levels in naturally occurring psychologic stresses. *Research Publications: Association for Research in Nervous and Mental Diseases,* 1962, 40 (23), 406-413.

Haurowitz, F. The foundations of immunology. In H. H. Fudenberg, D. P. Stites, J. L. Caldwell, & J. V. Wells (Eds.), *Basic & Clinical Immunology.* 3rd edition. Los Altos, California: Lange Medical Publications, 1980, 9-15.

Hirschhorn, K., Bach, R., Kolodny, R., Rirschein, I., & Hashem, N. Immune response and mitosis of human peripheral blood lymphocytes in vitro. *Science,* 1963 (3596), 142, 1185-1187.

Jenner, E. *An Inquiry into the Causes and Effects of the Variolae Vaccinae, a Disease Discovered in Some of the Western Counties of England, Particularly Gloucestershire, and Known by the Name of "the Cow Pox."* London: Sampson Low, 1798.

Köhler, G., & Milstein, C. Continuous cultures ot tused cells secreting antibody of predefined specificity. *Nature* (London), 1975, 256 (5517), 495-497.

Köhler, G., & Milstein, C. Derivation of specific antibody-producing tissue culture and tumor lines by cell fusion. *European Journal of Immunology,* 1976, 6 (7), 511-519.

Korneva, E. A., & Khai, L. M. On the role of the sympathoadrenal system in the regulation of the process of immunogenesis. *Fiziologicheskii Zhyrnal SSSR im I. M. Sechenova,* 1961, 47 (10), 1298-1305.

Korneva, E. A., & Khai, L. M. Effect of the stimulation of different mesencephalic structures on the course of immunological reactions. *Fizio-logicheskii Zhyrnal SSSR im I. M. Sechenova*, 1967, 53, 42-45. (in Russian)

Langman, R. E. The origin and significance of class discrimination in immunity. *Immunology Today*, 1984, 5(7), 194-196.

Leshan, L.L., & Worthington, R. E. Personality as factor in pathogenesis of cancer: Review of literature. *British Journal of Medical Psychology*, 1956, 29 (1), 49-56.

Lloyd, R. Mechanisms of psychoneuroimmunological response. In B. H. Fox & B. H. Newberry (Eds.), *Impact of Psychoendocrine Systems in Cancer and Immunity*. Toronto: C. J. Hogrefe, Inc., 1984a, 1-57.

Lloyd, R. Possible mechanisms of psychoneuroimmunological interaction. *Advances*, 1984b, 1, 43-51.

Malkovsky, M., & Medawar, P. B. Is immunological tolerance (non-responsiveness) a consequence of interleukin 2 deficit during the recognition of antigen? *Immunology Today*, 1984, 5 (12), 340-343.

Mandelbrote, B. M., & Wittkower, E. D. Emotional factors in Graves' disease. *Psychosomatic Medicine*, 1955, 17 (2), 109-117.

McClary, A. R., Meyer, E., & Weitzman, D. J. Observations on role of mechanism of depression in some patients with disseminated lupus erythematosus. *Psychosomatic Medicine*, 1965, 17 (4), 311-321.

Metal'nikov, S. *Rôle du Système Nerveux et des Facteurs Biologiques et Psychiques dans l'Immunité*. Paris: Masson, 1934. (in French)

Metal'nikov, S. & Chorine, V. Rôle des réflexes conditionnels dans l'immunité. *Annals de L'Institut Pasteur (Paris)*, 1926, 40 (11), 893-900. (in French)

Monjan, A. A. Stress and immunologic competence: Studies in animals. In R. Ader (Ed.), *Psychoneuroimmunology*. New York: Academic Press, 1981, 185-228.

Moos, R. H. Personality factors associated with rheumatoid arthritis: A review. *Journal of Chronic Diseases*, 1964, 17 (1), 41-55.

Moos, R. H., & Solomon, G. F. Psychologic comparisons between women with rheumatoid arthritis and their nonarthritic sisters. I. Personality test and interview rating data. *Psychosomatic Medicine*, 1965a, 27 (2), 135-149.

Moos, R. H., & Solomon, G. F. Psychologic comparisons between women with rheumatoid arthritis and their non-arthritic sisters. II. Content analysis of interviews. *Psychosomatic Medicine*, 1965b, 27 (2), 150-164.

Murray, J. B. New trends in psychosomatic research. *Genetic and Psychological Monographs*, 1977, 96, 3-74.

Pasteur, L. *Studies on Fermentation. The Diseases of Beer, Their Causes, and the Means of Preventing Them*. (A translation, made with the author's sanction, of *Études sur la Biére*; with notes, index, and original illustrations, by F. Faulkner & D. C. Robb.) London: MacMillan, 1879.

Rabkin, J. G., & Struening, E. L. Life events, stress and illness. *Science*, 1976,

194 (4269), 1013-1020.

Riley, V., Fitzmaurice, M. A., & Spackman, D. H. Psychoneuroimmunologic factors in neoplasia: Studies in animals. In R. Ader (Ed.), *Psychoneuroimmunology*. New York: Academic Press, 1981, 31-102.

Rosenberg, Y. J., Steinberg, A. D., & Santoro, T. J. The basis of autoimmunity in MRL-lpr/lpr mice: A role for self Ia-reactive T cells. *Immunology Today*, 1984, 5 (3), 64-67.

Scott, D. W. All self antigens are not created (tolerated) equally. *Immunology Today*, 1984, 5 (3), 68-69.

Selye, H. The general adaptation syndrome and the diseases of adaptation. *Journal of Clinical Endocrinology*, 1946, 6 (2), 117-230.

Shukla, H. C., Solomon, G. F., & Doshi, R. P. The relevance of some Ayurvedic (traditional Indian medical) concepts to modern holistic health. *Journal of Holistic Health*, 1979, 4, 125-131.

Silverstein, A. M. History of immunology. Cellular versus humoral immunity: Determinants and consequences of an epic 19th century battle. *Cellular Immunology*, 1979, 48 (1), 208-221.

Solomon, G. F. Emotional and personality factors in the onset and course of autoimmune disease, particularly rheumatoid arthritis. In R. Ader (Ed.), *Psychoneuroimmunology*. New York: Academic Press, 1981b, 159-182.

Solomon, G. F., & Amkraut, A. A. Psychoneuroendocrinological effects on the immune response. *Annual Review of Microbiology*, 1981, 35, 155-184.

Solomon, G. F., & Moos, R. H. Emotions, immunity, and disease: A speculative theoretical integration. *Archives of General Psychiatry*, 1964, 11 (6), 657-674.

Solomon, G. F., & Moos, R. H. The relationship of personality to the presence of rheumatoid factor in asymptomatic relatives of patients with rheumatoid arthritis. *Psychosomatic Medicine*, 1965, 27 (4), 350- 360.

Sorkin, E. Book review: Impact of Psychoendocrine Systems in Cancer and Immunity, edited by B. H. Fox, and B. H. Newberry. Toronto: C. J. Hogrefe, Inc., 1984. *Immunology Today*, 1984, 5 (9), 277-278.

Spector, N. H. The central state of the hypothalamus in health and disease: Old and new concepts. In P. J. Morgane & J. Panksepp (Eds.), *Handbook of the Hypothalamus. Physiology of the Hypothalamus*, Vol. 2. New York: Marcel Dekker, 1980, 453-517.

Spector, N. H., & Korneva, E. A. Neurophysiology, immunophysiology and neuroimmunomodulation. In R. Ader (Ed.), *Psychoneuroimmunology*. New York: Academic Press, 1981, 449-473.

Talal, N. *Autoimmunity: Genetic, Immunologic, Virologic and Clinical Aspects*. New York: Academic Press, 1977.

Talal, N. Autoimmunity and the immunologic network. *Arthritis and Rheumatism*, 1978, 21 (7), 858-861.

Talal, N. Autoimmunity. In H. H. Fudenberg, D. P. Stites, J. L. Caldwell, & J. V. Wells (Eds.), *Basic & Clinical Immunology*. 3rd edition. Los Altos, California: Lange Medical Publications, 1980, 220-231.

Theofilopoulos, A. N. Autoimmunity. In D. P. Stites, J. D. Stobo, H. H. Fudenberg, & J. V. Wells (Eds.), *Basic & Clinical Immunology*. 5th edition. Los Altos, California: Lange Medical Publications, 1984, 152-186.

Vessey, S. H. Effects of grouping on levels of circulating antibodies in mice. *Proceedings of the Society for Experimental Biology and Medicine*, 1964, 115 (1), 252-255.

Weiner, H. *Psychobiology and Human Disease*. New York: Elsevier, 1977.

Chapter 2

The Immune System

> I have become increasingly convinced that the essence
> of the immune system is the repression of its lymphocytes.
>
> Niels K. Jerne, *Towards a Network Theory*
> *of the Immune System,* 1974.

Our knowledge of cellular and molecular processes in immunity has ex-
ploded exponentially in the past two decades. To realize the dimensions of

the new knowledge, one need only peruse a standard 1950s era medical school textbook of microbiology (under which subject immunology was then subsumed) to come upon the single, terse comment: "The function of the lymphocyte is unknown"!

This present chapter is designed for behavioral scientists and physicians who completed graduate training before 1980! Our intention will be to present an abbreviated, somewhat simplified, but necessarily technical, introduction to the structural and functional characteristics of the immune system. The system is intricate, composed of numerous and diverse elements. To offset the likelihood, therefore, of presenting a rather fragmented account by describing each such element in turn, the chapter will carry an accompanying thread of clinical observations. By approaching the subject in this way, such immunologically-mediated conditions as autoimmune and immunodeficiency diseases, allergy, and tissue rejection can be understood in terms of relevant immune mechanisms. Furthermore, quite beyond their intrinsic interest, clinical examples should lend cohesion and depth to the discussion and help to clarify certain aspects of immune function whose description might otherwise verge on the abstract.

There are abstractions to be considered, nevertheless, that lend a particular interest to the story of immunology. One might ask, for example, if there are not attributes of "self," the "self" of our own self-knowledge, that translate to an immunologic frame of reference. Further, how does the immune system itself define the "self"? What is meant by immune specificity? by the concept of idiotypy? And why are these two concepts of any importance in understanding the workings of immunity? What constitutes immunologic memory? immunologic tolerance? Questions of this nature will, in a manner of speaking, form the backbone of this chapter by helping to support the few, among countless, details of immune system function selected for discussion.

The efficient, efficacious, and *appropriate* interaction of molecules and cells is, without doubt, the *sine qua non* of resilient immunologic defense. This being said, it is obvious that the immune system must carry on decision-making of a high order. In its confrontation with antigen (Gr., *anti*, against; *gen*, to create), or, in the event of altered "self" configuration, which cell class, or combination of classes, which molecular moiety, or constellation of molecules, will most likely carry the day? To quote from a recent article by Melvin Cohn: "In order to respond in an appropriate way to antigen the immune system must make two unavoidable decisions: the self-nonself discrimination, and the determination of effector class. Everything else follows from these considerations" (Cohn, 1985, p. 202).

As we shall see, much follows upon the choice of "effector class," for almost without exception, cells of the immune system act in concert, *in relationship* to one another. Rather than begin this review, therefore, with a sort of priority listing of these components, giving the more notable features of each, one by one, we will instead hope to convey a general idea of lymphocyte function (beyond what can be gained in the context of later discussion) by citing various examples of the interdependent behavior of these principal immune effector, regulatory, and accessory cells.

Immunologically competent cells have ways of speaking to one another that are rigorously precise, the precision (and uniqueness) of their language being derived, to an appreciable extent, from the separate loci that nurture their development: i.e., the microenvironments of the thymus gland, bone marrow, lymph nodes, and spleen. A general description of these organ and tissue sites will therefore be included as a part of this preliminary material. For reasons that will become clear as the text unfolds, there will be special emphasis placed on the microenvironment of the thymus.

WHY AN IMMUNE SYSTEM?

The ready answer to this question is obvious. The immune system is a defense system designed to protect the host on two fronts: it must protect from infective agents, without; from aberrance in self-structures, within. Much of this chapter will be devoted to elucidating these less-than-simple protective mechanisms.

At the outset, however, the question "why an immune system?" prompts other, rather more abstruse questions. What, for example, might be said of other dimensions of "self" protected by other, less tangible strategems of defense? When the idea of selfhood is examined at the relatively abstract level of human psychology—the self that evolves from a panoply of cognitive and emotional postures, subjectively elaborated and consolidated over time—is this transposition so very remote from our central theme? Does the term "self," when so considered, relate at all to immunity?

We are prepared to think of human personality as achieving definition through countless discriminations in thought and behavior, through conscious (and unconscious) recognition, recall, and choice based on the compatibility, commonality, or "rightness of fit" sensed in the general environment of life, the congress of one's fellow beings doubtless representing the most telling environment of all.

Do these perspectives on the self accommodate to a more strictly biological realm? Can they be comfortably introduced into an immunologic frame of reference? It would seem so. For, without doing violence to the concept, we find the lowliest unicellular organism generously equipped with a phagocytic immune repertoire that is primed for recognition, discrimination, and memorization—the very capacities most indispensable to its survival in the hostile microcosm. We find the vertebrates, as well as the most primitive of invertebrates, ready to utilize every possible mechanism to delimit the self, every effect of host-*versus*-other complementarity, or dissonance, brought continuously into full play. "Using one [allelochemical] signal or another, each form of life announces its proximity to the others around it, setting limits on encroachment or spreading welcome to potential symbionts." These words fittingly describe the adaptive ambivalence by which all living creatures, including human beings, protect and further themselves—and, not incidentally, enhance the "homeostasis of the earth"—by responding to discriminatory cues (Thomas, 1974, p. 41).

The immune system is an almost miraculous expression in all its operations of these same tendencies and vectors, attractions and repulsions, that must, in their sum, energize in defense of the integral "self" on the one hand, in abhorrence of the "alien" on the other. Also, by reason of its own intrinsic equilibrium, the immune system exhibits an essential characteristic of "organism as entity." It is this complicated dynamic of immune homeostasis, needless to say, that holds in check forces that are potentially destructive to the integrity of the host, the self.

THE CELLS, ORGANS, AND TISSUES OF IMMUNITY

The immune system is a widely dispersed matrix of organ and tissue sites for cell genesis and deposition, interconnected, perfused, and drained in its entirety by an arborization of lymphatic vessels. As mobile component of the system, a self-regulating network of white blood cells fine-tunes it to a steady state (Jerne, 1974), is ever-vigilant against the neoplastic transformation of somatic cells, and orchestrates appropriate immunologic response to such foreign particulate elements as viruses, mycobacteria, and fungi.

In addition, the immune system responds vigorously, in allogeneic reaction (Gr. *allos*, different), to within-species blood group antigens (alloantigens) introduced in blood transfusion, as well as to the transplantation of genetically incompatible organs and tissues. The opposite circumstance, elicited in response to allogeneic lymphoid tissue and/or cell transplantation—as seen, for example, in the graft-versus-host reaction, wherein activated immune cells within a graft attack host tissue (Deeg &

Storb, 1984)—testifies to the fact that the immune system is not an infal-
lible defense against external insult.

Normal Patterns of Cell Communication

In 1966, Claman, Chaperon, and Triplett conducted a group of experiments on lethally irradiated 9- to 12-week-old mice, first introducing
cell suspensions of thymocytes, then adding suspensions of bone marrow
cells to offset the deleterious effects of radiation on erythromyelopoiesis.
The animals were challenged with sheep erythrocytes, sacrificed, and their
spleens excised for analysis of hemolytic foci under each of the three separate conditions: injection of thymocytes alone, bone marrow cells alone,
and a mixed suspension of the two. Thus, through experiments initially
designed solely "to test for the existence of potentially immunocompetent
cells in the thymus" (p. 1167), the discovery was made that thymus and
marrow cells had the greater stimulatory effect on spleen hemolysis when
acting in combination. Not knowing, in absolute certainty, which cell type
might be responsible for which function, "effector" or "auxiliary," Claman
and his colleagues nonetheless correctly presumed the two cell types to be
functionally specific. This single experiment ushered in a fertile period of
experimentation, one that has not diminished in intensity to this day.

Early work was largely devoted to identifying those elements of the
immune complex responsible for the production of antibody—experiments
on the immunologic consequences of spleen and thymus extirpation in
laboratory animals showing the way. The nature of the interaction between
classes of lymphocytic cells (B and T lymphocytes) in antibody production soon became a subject of equal interest, for interact they must, in
view of the fact that neonatal thymectomy was proven to lead to a complete absence of circulating antibody (Miller, 1962).

Today, there is general agreement that the transformation of B lymphocytes to antibody-secreting cells is a sequential, three-stage process
that is dependent upon T lymphocytes: a stage of activation (receptor induction), one of growth and proliferation, and one of differentiation
(maturation). These stages are discrete and have been shown to be selectively stimulated and enhanced by soluble molecular products of the T
lymphocyte known as lymphokines (Rocklin, Bendtzen, & Greineder,
1980). For example, growth and proliferation are mediated by the lymphokine, B cell growth factor (BCGF), whereas differentiation requires the
presence of the lymphokine, B cell differentiation factor (BCDF)—although the separateness of function here may not be absolute (Kishimoto,
1985). Given the fact that some of the most devastating afflictions, such as

the malignant lymphomas and myelomas, are characterized by serum immunoglobulin excess, first attempts are underway at utilizing these potent regulatory molecules in specific therapies for a variety of lymphoproliferative disorders, including specific immunologic deficiencies (Goldstein & Chiragos, 1981; Lane et al., 1984; Oldham, 1982).

Abnormal Patterns of Cell Communication

An area of abiding interest in immunology has been the patterns of communication defined by leukocytes and their accessory cells. What intrinsic forces power this regulatory circuitry? How prominent a regulatory role do "auxiliary" cells play therein? What of T cell subsets? What fine adjustments in immune regulation allow, in normal homeostasis, for a balance of helper *versus* suppressor activity? If, as happens in certain disease states, that balance becomes disturbed, in what respect is the disturbance manifested, and by what mechanism is it brought about? If, as in the antibody-deficient condition, acquired hypogammaglobulinemia, the immune defect is not intrinsic to B cells (which it is not), does the abnormality rest with a relative helper T cell deficiency, or with excessive suppressor T cell activity (Katz, 1984)?

In fact, answers to some of these questions are at hand, and some rather clear-cut relationships are being drawn with respect to immune regulation and disease process. The generality holds, first of all, that immune system disequilibrium and disease can be mutually associated phenomena. The use of monoclonal antibodies (i.e., identical, replicate antibodies of exquisite sensitivity) in both fundamental research and clinical diagnosis and therapy has helped to establish this one important relationship. However, it should come as no surprise that the disconcerting question of cause and effect awaits untangling.

In more specific terms, *patterns* of relationship are holding as well. For it is now evident that a principal basis for immune system imbalance rests with deviations from an optimal ratio of regulatory lymphocytes: namely, an optimal ratio between T helper or T_4 cells, and T suppressor or T_8 cells (T_4/T_8 ratio). For example, a diminution in circulating T suppressor (T_8) cells is a characteristic of the neurological disease, multiple sclerosis (MS), circulating suppressor lymphocytes being significantly decreased in number during acute phases of the disease, only to reappear during times of remission. The rheumatic autoimmune disorder, systemic lupus erythematosus (SLE), is also characterized by a loss of function in suppressor circuits. By contrast, the acquired immunodeficiency syndrome (AIDS) is a condition characterized by an abnormally low T_4/T_8 ratio

(Lane & Fauci, 1985). Depending on the clinical condition under study, "loss" of circulating T lymphocytes has been attributed to cell sequestration in particular tissue compartments, to the the the presence of antibody cytotoxic to T lymphocytes (see Hauser & Weiner, 1984; McFarlin, 1984; Morimoto, et al., 1980, for recent reviews), or, as in the case of AIDS, to the selective destruction by virus of the T helper cell subset (Fauci et al., 1985).

Microenvironments in Lymphoid Organs

The lymphatic vessels form an encompassing loop, joining *efferent* lymph channels to the thoracic and right lymphatic ducts, these larger, collecting channels then directing both blood and lymph through the vena cava to the right, receiving chamber of the heart. Within the arterial circulation, lymph (a filtrate of blood plasma) moves, once again, in its *afferent* pathway, into the extracellular tissue spaces, and thence into strategically positioned secondary lymphoid organs and aggregations. Stated more precisely, the peripheral lymph channels transport processed antigen, cellular detritus, macrophages, plasma cells, and a continuously recirculating pool of viable, antigen-primed lymphocytes from sites of entrapment, the spleen and lymph nodes, into the efferent limb of the arc, and so to the heart. Microscopic lymph capillaries, distributed throughout all tissues of the body (excepting brain, eye, and spinal cord), initiate this passage, and the spleen (as a filter of blood) and lymph nodes (as filters of lymph) act as all-important way stations along this circuit. The thymus gland lies outside the circuit, in the sense that it is solely a source of migratory thymocytes destined for occupancy of the lymph nodes and spleen, but does not function as a filter.

The Thymus Gland

The two functional arms of the immune system, cellular and humoral, are mutually, but not similarly, dependent upon its principal organ, the thymus gland. Through mechanisms that have yet to be satisfactorily defined, the internal environment of the gland has a direct influence on the early development of one of the two principal classes of lymphocytes, the T cells. By means of the aforementioned molecules, the lymphokines (Pick, 1984), the regulatory subclass of T_4 (helper) cells communicates with, and controls, in turn, the early development of B lymphocytes, as well as the activities of that highly purposeful member of the phagocyte class, the macrophage. Thus, both by direction and indirection, the thymus regulates and controls the more important effector systems of immunity.

In addition, the endocrine thymus profoundly affects various vital functions of the body, other than immunity. By way of illustration, severe immunodeficiency in infants, or a state of athymia in laboratory animals, are both inevitably associated with a failure to thrive, runting, an inability to reject allograft, and the likelihood of early death. Total thymic aplasia, as seen in the Di George syndrome (Conley et al, 1979), will result in complete absence of circulating antibody, whereas in the somewhat less radical condition of cellular immunodeficiency, in which a remnant of thymic tissue remains (Nezeldof's syndrome), serum immunoglobulins will approach near-normal levels (Buckley, 1982).

The thymus is a bilobed structure of primitive pharyngeal origin. Each of its lobes is comprised of an outermost capsule, a subcapsular cortex, an inner cortex, and a central medulla. In essence, the gland is a mass of lymphocytes that is supported and compartmentalized by a delicate, penetrable reticular infrastructure. Within these matrices, populations of T lymphoblasts, both stable and transient, coexist in various stages of maturation and differentiation.

As early as the ninth week of gestation, the cortex of the thymus gland is colonized by large, immunologically incompetent lymphoblasts, the progeny of primitive, lymphoid stem cells that have migrated through the bloodstream to the developing thymic epithelium from the bone marrow, their locus of origin (Lajtha, 1979). The thymic cortex then becomes a primary site of both lymphocytopoiesis and cell death. It is of interest to note here that these same stem cells of the bone marrow themselves play a part in bringing about the full maturation of the epithelium of the thymus (Pahwa, Pahwa, & Good, 1978).

Within a matter of hours, and in substantially reduced numbers, the juvenile T cells move through the cortical interstices into the medulla of the gland. Once in association with this particular epithelial stroma, and preliminary to their emigration (ecotaxis) as "virgin lymphocytes" to predefined areas of the spleen and lymph nodes, the surviving lymphoblasts continue to undergo a process of differentiation that, although antigen-*independent*, will nevertheless result in the development of several T cell lines of differing functional capacity (i.e., memory cells, helper, and suppressor/cytotoxic cells) (Cantor & Boyse, 1975).

It is thought that this secondary stage of differentiation within the thymus occurs under the influence of a number of low-molecular-weight polypeptide hormones secreted by the epithelial cells of the gland (Bach et al., 1979; Goldstein et al., 1978). Distinguishing T cell surface molecules develop into their more mature (but not necessarily final) form during this time, marking an event that will become critically important to immune cell intercommunication (Reinherz & Schlossman, 1980). For example, the "helper" signal specialization, which now appears on the surface coat of a majority of thymocytes destined to become the T_4 subset, will activate small, quiescent B lymphocytes into blastosis and the production of plasma cells; in reverse effect, the "suppressor" signal, displayed on the outer membrane of the T_8 subset, will diminish B cell function.

One of the most important aspects of the thymic "education" of the lymphocyte has to do with the fact that each of these specializations is elaborated in an histo-(tissue) compatibility context. In other words, it is not until they have been exposed to the histocompatibility phenotype of both the thymic cortical and medullary epithelia that thymocytes become mature, immunologically competent cells (Bhan et al., 1980; Haynes, 1984). As a result of such exposure, this particular cell class is imparted an imprimatur of "self" that can only benefit the immunologic defense and adaptive endowment of the host (Benacerraf, 1981).

In a striking demonstration of thymic impact on immune cell ontogeny, Kruisbeek et al. (1981) have shown that cytotoxic T lymphocyte (CTL) precursor cells from congenitally athymic ("nude") mice are developmentally restricted by the particular tissue compatible characteristics of engrafted semi- and fully-allogeneic (nonself) neonatal thymic tissue. To quote from the summary statement in this paper: it is "the MHC (major histocompatibility complex) phenotype of the intrathymic environment that dictates which MHC determinants the CTL precursors differentiating within it will specifically recognize as self-determinants" (p. 2175).

Deserving emphasis in this very brief resumé is the role performed by the "skin immune system" (Bos & Kapsenberg, 1986) in thymocyte maturation. There is mounting evidence that keratinocytes, cells of the basal layer of the epidermis, produce a substance very like, if not identical to, the thymic hormone, thymopoietin. In addition, an immune associated (Ia) histocompatibility molecule has been detected on the surface membranes of both keratinocytes and Langerhans' cells in skin. The hypothesis has been put forward, therefore, that these particular cells may indeed constitute "an integral component of the human immune system," and that they may be essential in affecting the full maturation of newly-evolved T lymphocytes upon their egress from the thymus gland (Edelson & Fink, 1985, p. 50). Two facts warrant mention here, as parenthetical note: (1) the epidermal Langerhans' cell line originates in bone marrow (Katz, Tamaki, & Sachs, 1979); (2) T cells themselves originate, during embryogenesis, from epithelial, rather than mesenchymal, tissue (Auerbach, 1961).

To summarize: by means of its milieu (hormonal or otherwise), the thymus gland imposes a characteristic cell surface antigenicity on T lymphocytes prior to their release, this phenotype predetermining a particular effector or regulatory role. In addition, this same milieu stimulates the development of recognition molecules for self-*versus*-nonself discrimination. The "nursing cells" of the thymus gland bestow (in a manner yet unclear) a capacity for histocompatibility pattern recognition on incipient T cell subpopulations (Stobo, 1984), and it has thus been inferred that there must exist environmental factors, intrinsic to the epithelial strata of the gland, that can effectuate the genetic rearrangements essential to the formulation of the various protein receptor specificities subserving recognition. Further, it is thought that these factors probably derive from the specialized cell coat molecules that configure the genetic determinants of histocompatibility, the so-called "determinants of self." The thymus fulfills these two important functions in the neonatal period on a long-lived population of cells that is presumed capable of survival throughout the lifespan of the organism (Smith, 1984).

As a final note, there is provocative evidence to show that the gland may not act alone in its important work. A picture of functional collaboration, involving both hormonal and histocompatibility effects, between the thymus gland and specific cells of the epidermis is presently evolving. In this proposed schema, certain epidermal cells are seen as contributing, in a supplemental, but essential, capacity, to the full immunocompetence of thymus-derived lymphocytes, *exclusively*, the B lymphocyte class being in no way directly affected by either skin or thymus.

The Spleen and Lymph Nodes

In contrast to the thymus, the two secondary organs of the immune system, the lymph nodes and spleen, are the two principal systemic sites of microbial and particulate filtration and entrapment. Herein, partially differentiated, "committed" T and B lymphocytes undergo further differentiation upon exposure to antigen, doing so in anatomically separate loci: in the lymph node, for example, B cells home to subcapsular germinal centers; T cells to germinal centers embedded within the diffuse nodular cortex. Other repository sites that fulfill much the same immunologic purpose as the nodes and spleen include the appendix, the pharynx (tonsils and adenoids), Peyer's patches in the small intestine, and the submucosal tissue of the genitourinary tracts and bronchia. From the point of view of immune protection, the favorable logistics of this tissue distribution are obvious, the epithelial tissue lining the lungs and the several tracts representing a locus that is relatively vulnerable to incursion by environmental pathogens.

In the lymph node, a recirculating pool of lymphocytes pass from blood to lymph, and back again, by either one of two routes: the first, by way of invagination through the cuboidal epithelial cells of postcapillary venules in the lymph node cortex; the second, by way of afferent and efferent lymphatic vessels that traverse the node. In the spleen, blood circulates through venous sinuses from splenic artery to splenic vein, and thence to the hepatic portal vein. The entrapment and processing of foreign matter carried within the arterial flow takes place at the conflux of afferent and efferent channels in the marginal zone of the red pulp. The pattern of splenic circulation dictates that macrophages of the red pulp prime the leukocyte populations that colonize the white pulp. Aside from its importance as "a large, discriminating filter set across the bloodstream" (Cooper, 1982, p. 248), the spleen is a blood reservoir and a major site of T and B lymphocyte production.

SOME FUNDAMENTAL CHARACTERISTICS OF IMMUNITY

Immune Specificity

The immune system demonstrates wide variation in the attribute of specificity. In general, it may be said to be both *specific* and *nonspecific* in its manner of operation. It will be seen, however, that independently developed immune cell groups show considerable functional overlap with respect to one or the other of these two operating modes.

The immune system is equipped to respond to a virtually limitless number and variety of invasive macromolecules (bacteria, viruses, proteins, complex polysaccharides, etc.) with *specific* powers of recognition and molecular binding by activated, cooperating colonies of preprogrammed lymphocytes; and to respond *nonspecifically* to tumor cells, extracellular debris, invading microbes, and parasitic organisms through the scavenging activities of phagocytic cells. Specific immunity is expressed in two wholly contrasting (but nonetheless interdependent) ways by two morphologically similar, but functionally distinct, populations of lymphocytes, the T and B cells. The processes of nonspecific immunity, on the other hand, are mediated by cells of the erythromyeloid series, a group that includes, apart from the erythrocytes, the phagocytes and kindred mediator cells.

The distinction between specific and nonspecific immunity is reflected in the divergent pathways of immune cell ontogeny. All cells of the immune system descend from undifferentiated, "pluripotential" stem cells, which make their way from the fetal liver to cloistered perivascular compartments in bone marrow in the second trimester of embryonic life. Herein, the ancestral cell divides, generating two cell lines, the lymphopoietic and the hemopoietic. Lymphopoietic stem cells become precursors to the lymphocyte series, of which B and T cells constitute the two principal cell classes. Hemopoietic stem cells are precursors to four cell types: erythrocytes, phagocytes (i.e., polymorphonuclear leukocytes, mononuclear macrophages, neutrophils, and eosinophils), motile basophils, and the nonmotile cells of connective tissue, the mast cells.

Although not always easily distinguishable in their gross morphology (particularly in preimmune quiescence), primed, immunocompetent T and B lymphocytes can be differentiated unambiguously on the basis of cell surface receptor conformation and function (Katz, 1977). As will be seen, T cells operate as effector and regulatory agents in specific, *cellular, or cell-mediated immunity*, whereas B lymphocytes are effector cells for specific, *humoral*, or *antibody-mediated, immunity*. A second important point of contrast between the two groups lies in their differing relationship to the thymus gland, the principal lymphoid organ.

That the distinction between specific and nonspecific immunologic mediation is by no means absolute is illustrated in the activities of one member of the phagocytic cell group, the macrophage. The capacities of this interesting cell are in fact pivotal to the sequential expression, first, of nonspecific, then specific, immunity. Hence, by its initial *nonspecific* attachment to an invading microbe, partial ingestion of same, subsequent release of products stimulatory to the lymphocyte (monokines), and ultimate "presentation" of antigen to the lymphocyte, the macrophage prepares the stage for T and B cell multiplication and differentiation. In so doing, it has of course initiated the specific end-phase of an immunologic response.

Specificity in T Lymphocytes

The majority of T cells are long-lived and highly mobile, typically circulating and recirculating—tirelessly "on patrol"—throughout the lymphatic and peripheral channels of the body. This surveillance also encompasses the brain to a limited extent, despite the presence of the blood-brain barrier and the absence of lymphatics in brain. The total population of T cells is characterized by a number of functional specializations acquired during its passage through the epithelial strata of the thymus gland, the effects of this passage thereafter differentiating T, or thymus-dependent lymphocytes, from B cells, or bone marrow-derived lymphocytes. Otherwise stated, the thymus gland exerts its influence on T lymphoblasts in such a way as to favor the development of several subsets within the T cells class. Each subset is uniquely coded for its specific biologic purpose by integral protein configurations on the surface coats of individual cells within the subset, each such configuration being specific to that subset: hence, the appellations, T helper/inducer cell, or T_4; T suppressor cell, or T_8; and T cytotoxic cell (CTL), or T_5. (Unambiguous distinction between T_8 and T_5 cell lines has yet to be established.)

Specificity in B Lymphocytes

B cells progress through a series of developmental steps of even greater complexity, but unlike T lymphocytes, do so in complete independencefrom thymic influence (albeit dependence upon T cell intermediation) (Honjo, 1983; Wall & Kuehl, 1983). Additionally, B cells, in contrast to T cells, are, in a sense, the indirect, rather than direct, mediators of humoral immunity, for it is their giant progeny, the plasma cells, not the antigen-primed parent B cell, that secrete antibodies, the proteins molecules that are destined to cross-link with antigen. The remarkable specificity *and* universality of antibody linkage, or binding, has remained a fascinating and challenging area of exploration in immunology since the turn of the century, dating, that is, from the *side chain theory* of antibody production proposed by Paul Ehrlich (1900).

Specificity in Mononuclear Phagocytic Cells

In contrast to the manifold ways in which T and B lymphocytes first encounter, then process, antigen, the endocytosis and intracellular digestion of foreign materials by cells of hemopoietic lineage is relatively non-specific and indiscriminant. The macrophage, for example, is formidably equipped for anti-infectious defense, as well as defense against the presence of transformed body cells, with an intracellular arsenal of more than 75 microbicidal and tumoricidal substances, its capacity for signal detection enabled by more than 30 plasma membrane receptor projections (Nathan & Cohn, 1985)! Yet, its unerring ability to home to target involves a process of "broad-specificity recognition" that, to date, remains imperfectly understood (Wilkinson, 1983).

Until such understanding comes about, it is generally acknowledged that the macrophage is lacking in specific powers of recognition and memory, at least as such powers are seen to govern the activities of the lymphopoietic cell line. Morover, its retention at the site of bacterial infiltration, as well as the limits of its activity while so retained, are both largely controlled by activating, inhibiting, and chemotactic molecules (lymphokines) secreted by sensitized lymphocytes (Adams & Hamilton, 1984; Dumond & Hamblin, 1983).

Phagocytosis is nonetheless a primitive immmune defense mechanism that has survived in all living organisms throughout phylogeny, from amoeba to sea urchin to Man. Moreover, aside from their efficacy—as may be imagined, given their formidable equipment—the mechanisms of defense mounted by cells of the hemopoietic series can be devastating in their impact. Mast cells, for example, produce the vasoactive substance, histamine, which brings about the immediate hypersensitivity, or systemic anaphylactic, response to specific protein allergen. Acute, spontaneous anaphylaxis is life-threatening. By affecting the respiratory and gastrointestinal tracts, the peripheral circulation and the heart, its sudden onset and rapid course can bring about bronchiolar and laryngeal spasm, gastrointestinal hypermotility (tenesmus), edema of the heart muscle and circulatory collapse, with ensuing coma and fatal shock.

Further Thoughts on Specificity

The term *specificity* has broad meaning in immunology. As a kind of first principle, it should be pointed out that an antigen is immunogenic only to the extent to which its molecular conformation has relative specificity for one, from a presumed assortment, of "recognition molecules" on the lymphocyte surface coat. A second interesting aspect of immune specificity is one that would seem to refute common sense: the simple—and somehow extraordinary—fact that the afferent limb of the immune system is unquestionably under "antigen drive." Thus, in a scenario that is at last becoming better understood, presenting antigen first seeks, then "recognizes," a like image in the conformation of preexisting elements within the defense system of the presumptive host! A vital stimulus to antigenicity apparently resides, therefore, not in any "template," or instructional, properties of antigen, as was long presumed (Breinl & Haurowitz, 1930; Haurowitz, 1970), but rather in the selective pattern recognition capability of the invasive macromolecule itself. To quote from N. K. Jerne's remarkable treatise on the integrative and regulatory capacities of immune cell networks: "the conclusion [seems] to be inescapable, that the antigen must bring into the cell information concerning the complementary structure of the antibody molecule" (Jerne, 1974, p. 37).

Recognition works both ways, however. Antigen specificity for membrane components of the lymphocyte determines, in turn, the degree of "avidity" for antigen expressed by the lymphocyte, a near-perfect fit between the molecular surface patterns of the two indicating what is known as "stereocomplementarity." This property is, by consequence, the most important determinant of specificity, and is the condition from which all else follows. Complementarity, and the degree of specificity it engenders, is fundamental, on the one hand, to the recognitive properties invested in the structure and chemistry of both the antigenic determinant (*epitope*) and the preimmune lymphocyte receptor molecule (*paratope*). On the other hand, ligand/receptor complementarity sets in motion the physicochemical forces that are essential for antigen binding (Leslie & Cohen, 1973).

The Repercussions of Binding

Antigenic determinant, marker, receptor, recognition molecule—terms of this sort are descriptors for the plasma membrane specializations through which cells communicate with one another. They are code vehicles for inductive biological process, are essential for intra- and inter-system information exchange, and are consequently generalizable across systems. They are as common, that is to say, to permutations in the receptor protein of pre- and postsynaptic nerve terminals during the transmission of nerve impulse as to the structural alterations accompanying the coupling of ligand (antigen) and receptor at the exterior surface of lymphocytes.

From this strategic position, antigen-specific receptor molecules bind to microorganisms and foreign molecules to form an antigen-receptor complex. As the initial event in signal transduction, binding elicits a series of cellular perturbations (phospholipid methylation, enzyme activation, receptor aggregation, calcium influx, and so forth) from surface membrane to nucleus.

In humoral immunity, the more obvious "down-stream" repercussions to binding divide into three principal phases: one, the proliferation of a B cell clone expressing membrane-bound immunoglobulin; two, the differentiation of B cell to plasmablast; and three, the secretion of free, monospecific antibodies into the lymphatic circulation by the mature plasma cell. In cellular immunity, to cite a single example, the surface-bound stimulus of target adhesion triggers cytotoxic T lymphocytes and the large granular lymphocytes known as natural killer (NK) cells to carry out lysis through the secretion of lysosomal enzymes from cytoplasmic granules, the appointed function of the cell (in this instance, granule exocytosis and the "lethal hit") again being calcium-dependent (Henkart, 1985; Hiserodt, Britvan, & Targan, 1982; Plaut, Bubbers, & Henney, 1976).

The Specificity of Idiotype

Antigen-antibody specificity—or, to put it more precisely, *individual* specificity—characterizes the encounter between a given organism and a given external antigen. It may be assumed that the genetic constitution and previous history of the organism have much to do with the intensity and outcome of the encounter, as well as its uniqueness. Such is the view that has predated the "paradigm shift" that is currently taking place in immunology. The new perspective would redefine the immune system as an internally-, rather than externally-directed, system. In brief, the immune system is now seen as chiefly relying for its integrity upon *receptor*, rather than antigen, specificity (Bona, 1984). According to this new understanding, antigen drives the system only to the extent to which it focuses and coordinates the activities of normally dissociated T and B cell clones. Antigen-specific immune responses are thus relegated to a secondary role, to what is described as "'accidents de parcours' in the life of an immune system" (Vaz, Martinez-A., & Coutinho, 1984, p. 44). The principal focus of attention is now directed upon *idiotype* (Kunkel, Mannick, & Williams, 1963; Oudin & Michel, 1963), for in *its* specificity, immunologists see an important clue to the riddle of immune regulation. They see, too, ways in which defects in the regulatory circuits of idiotypes might be amenable to manipulation in specific therapies (Kennedy, Melnick, & Dreesman, 1986).

Idiotypes are receptors. More precisely, they are chemical structures ("determinants") present in the hypervariable regions of particular domains (V domains) located within the side-arm polypeptide chains of immunoglobulin molecules. According to the present view, the role of the idiotype (and consequently that of the antibody molecule on which it appears) is two-fold. An idiotype not only constitutes a recognition and combining site for antigen, but is *itself* immunogenic: i.e., an idiotype can act both as structural mirror image to antigen, and as *internal* antigen, or self-epitope, for antibody (Burnet, 1978; Jerne, 1974).

This remarkable state of affairs can be explained in terms of feedback inhibition. Once the number of antibodies raised against specific antigen exceeds a critical threshold during the proliferative response of the stimulated lymphocyte, sets of such determinants (*idiotopes*) presented on multiple antibody molecules and T cell-bound receptors will elicit the production of still another set of *antiidiotypic antibodies* of comparable specificity, these latter receptors, raised to a optimal concentration, then being capable of stimulating anti-antiidiotypes, and so on.

The process is circular, involuted, and self-referenced, in the sense that it allows for internal control. Stimulatory (T cell help) and inhibitory (T cell suppression) feedback are selectively activated, and so exert a fine control over the clonal proliferation of effector cells (Eardley et al., 1978).

Other internal loops operate through a circuitry of shared idiotypic specificity that may *or may not* be directly linked to the particular specificity of the initiating antigen (Oudin & Casenave, 1971). Perhaps most important, each of these elements of control favors the attainment of ever-changing, adaptive states of equilibrium (Jerne, 1974). (It will perhaps not have escaped notice here that the end result of idiotypic-antiidiotypic interaction is not dissimilar to the effects of down-regulation observed in peptide hormonal systems, whereby receptor number is subject to intrinsic influence, again in the interests of homeostasis [King & Cuatrecasas, 1981; Pastan & Willingham, 1981]).

Summary

The concept of idiotypy therefore implies unceasing discourse between signal and receptor units throughout all physiologic systems, perpetuated always in relation to the external world. "If one agrees that idiotypes may sterically represent mirror images of antigens, it would be reasonable to suppose that the immune system accepts the structural diversity in the universe as nothing new or strange since it 'sees' these structures continuously in its complementary circuits" (Theofilopoulos, 1984, p. 162). Now, more than 20 years following their discovery, idiotypes are helping to explain those special attributes of the immune system that have been so long a source of wonder: its plasticity, its extreme diversity, and its extraordinary recognitive capacities. Moreover, it is presumed that the stability of the system—maintained in constancy despite constant change—must necessarily profoundly affect the equilibrium of the internal universe entire, the two equilibria being integral, one to the other (Vaz et al., 1984).

The contribution of genes to this entire process constitutes a tale unto itself. It is nevertheless germane to this present discussion to note that the specificity for immunogen demonstrated by the immunoglobulin receptor (and, eventually, by free antibody) has been found to be genetically controlled, this control exerting itself by combinations of gene segments positioned (as are idiotypes) either within, or contiguous to, the hypervariable domain of the immunoglobulin molecule. Of considerable interest in this regard is the finding that the random mutation and translocation of these gene clusters not only operate in the somatic development of the several immune cell repertoires—which is, of course, to be expected—but that these same processes also prevail throughout the duration of an immune response, providing, thereby, a fascinating example of Darwinian evolution in microcosm (Manser et al., 1985).

Memory in Immunity

Structural specificity and complementarity are aspects of histocompatibility gene composition that characterize the uniquely encoded immune systems of individual organisms, allowing for the "demarcation of individuality" (Vaz et al., 1984). These two properties also act as primary antigen-associated stimuli to lymphoid cell differentiation upon initial exposure of an organism to antigen (primary response), and as selective vehicles for the exponential proliferation (1000-fold!) of lymphocyte clones from lymphoblasts and antibody-producing plasma cells upon subsequent exposure (secondary, or anamnestic, response) (Katz, 1977; Marchalonis, 1976).

Recognition molecules on the lymphoid cell membrane carry the latent morphological residuals of immunologic memory. For example, the so-called memory cells of the B cell class constitute a small, select group of long-lived lymphocytes, descendants of a second daughter cell line (the antibody-producing plasmacyte representing the first). Both B cell lineages are capable of synthesizing, and of secreting into the circulation, immunoglobulin molecules with binding structures identical to the original recognition glycoproteins found on the surface membranes of parent cells. It also follows that each of these familially-related molecules shares an identical specificity for the inducing antigen (Burnet, 1959).

At the time of first challenge by antigen, the specificity of the encounter undergoes incorporation at the molecular level in B precursor cells, this specificity retaining its stamp throughout each maturational stage of B cell development, until, at terminal stage, plasma cells actively secrete antigen-specific immunoglobulin. The immune system is now "primed."

The best morphologic evidence of this transformation is the appearance of germinal follicles in the marginal zone of the spleen, areas that serve as an "amplification system" for the progressive selection of antigen-reactive lymphocyte clones, as well as encapsulated arenas for the proliferation of memory B and T cells. Thus primed, the immune system will respond with greater rapidity and with more robust production of antibody upon subsequent challenge than at the time of initial antibody induction (Cooper, 1982).

Tolerance in Immunity

Given its phenomenal powers of surveillance, and the obvious ease with which it generates reactive antibody, how, it might be asked, does the immune system acquire a tolerance, or "unresponsiveness," to structures of the "self?" The question is basic to an understanding of immunity, and has stimulated intense study and theoretical debate over the past 40 years, beginning with the observations of Owen (1945) on the unexpected presence of histo*incompatible* blood cells in dizygotic bovine twins.

Apart from unravelling the mechanism(s) of induced tolerance to organ and tissue allograft (Billingham, Brent, & Medawar, 1953; Brent, 1981; French & Batchelor, 1969), there have been two crucial questions relating to tolerance. First of all, how is the state of unresponsiveness to autoantigens during fetal and neonatal life (Burnet & Fenner, 1949) to be explained? Second, what alterations in immune status can account for the release from the constraints of self-tolerance that occurs in chronic diseases of autoimmunity in adult organisms (Theofilopoulos, 1984)? Maternal tolerance to trophoblast in pregnancy has been still another intriguing aspect of tolerance under study (Faulk & McIntyre, 1981). The condition is the more intriguing when it is shown that, despite the presence of so-called "maternal blocking factors" (Rocklin et al., 1976), maternal recognition of, and immunity to, the fetal-placental unit may be a relatively common, though benign, occurrence in normal pregnancy (Faulk & Johnson, 1977; O'Sullivan et al., 1982).

In essence, working hypotheses on the subject of tolerance do not differ significantly in their central point from the first investigations of acquired immunologic tolerance carried out in the 1950s, researches for which Sir MacFarlane Burnet and Sir Peter B. Medawar shared the Nobel Prize in Physiology and Medicine (1960). It is now understood that the immature immune system characteristically demonstrates tolerance (principally mediated by the B cell compartment) within a narrow "window" (Brent et al., 1976) in the perinatal period, a period that has been described as an "obligatory paralyzable phase" (Nossal & Pike, 1980). This special condition appears, incidentally, to be as true of select subsets of lymphocytes during all life stages, neonatal and adult, as of the immature immune system as a whole.

As might be expected, given the foregoing discussion on the importance of receptor activation to the viability of cells, possible mechanisms of tolerance under consideration and experimental test have included receptor blockade, receptor "freeze," receptor endocytosis and shedding, and the inhibition of immunoglobulin synthesis. Inasmuch as immune tolerance evidently results from the incorporation—and perpetuation—of a negative signal at the most fundamental, molecular level, it is thought likely that some part of the receptor complement presented by "natural" suppressor (NS) cells of the neonatal spleen (Strober, 1984) plays an important role in tolerance induction (Dorf & Benacerraf, 1984; Nossal, 1983).

THE GENETICS OF IMMUNITY

Unquestionably, a deeper understanding of the link between genes and immunity will result from continued basic research on the molecular recognition structures responsible for protecting histocompatibility. Needless to say, the physiology and biophysics of the cell receptors that incorporate these structures have become matters of great intrinsic interest to biological science.

Of no less importance, however, has been the realization that receptor conformation can convey information of comparable *clinical* interest. It has been suggested, for example, that should synthetic immunogenic technology be directed, in an interdisciplinary effort, to a focal point of convergence between body systems (namely, the cell surface receptor and its complementary anti-receptor structure), answers might be forthcoming to a crucial question in medicine: why, in certain disease states, do the "boundary zones" dividing these systems break down, zones that normally remain strictly delimited? (Köhler, 1980).

Dating from the discovery of the major histocompatibility complex (MHC), there is no doubt that the differentiation of immune cell types into distinct functional subgroups, as well as the interaction of these groups, are critical aspects of immune responsivity carried out under varying degrees of genetic control, or "restriction." For the sake of clarity, therefore, if not simplicity—given the complexity of the topic—it would seem useful to describe some of the principal features of immunity from the perspective of genetics. Our purpose herein will be to convey an overall impression of these immutable forces that imbue the immune system with an impressive degree of autonomy.

Furthermore, in a book that argues for the importance of attitudinal and behavioral variables in influencing the onset and course of disease, it should be borne in mind throughout that compelling evidence now exists to support the premise that a predisposition to any one of several chronic diseases (including a number of autoimmune disorders) is genetically preprogrammed in particular individuals. In other words, individual differences in immune responsivity exist in association with specific antigenic histocompatibility phenotypes. In sum, the advent of DNA analysis and recombinant DNA cloning technology, the clinical procedure of tissue typing, and the diagnostic and therapeutic use of monoclonal antibodies have brought a wealth of new information to the fore that has made cognizance of genetic disease predisposition inescapable.

The Major Histocompatibility Complex (MHC)

The immune system has been described as a "microcosmos," a self-contained, self-directing network of cells with a seemingly boundless capacity to "create a mirror image of all structures in the universe" (Köhler, Levitt, & Bach, 1981, p. 58). This ability to recognize and to discriminate between autologous (self) and foreign molecules, as well as to coordinate the selective differentiation and interaction of heterogeneous populations of lymphocytic and phagocytic cells, attests to inherent mechanisms of control. Some of the genetically determined molecules responsible for the mediation of histocompatibility are instrumental in protecting self-identity. Still others serve to initiate and regulate immune system response to antigen incursion—not alone response, but appropriateness of response (Dausset, 1981).

A general picture of the mechanisms of immune system autonomy has evolved from the study of clusters of genes, distinct to particular chromosomal loci, which code for transmembranous glycoprotein structures on virtually all nucleated body cells. Thus widely distributed, alloantigens help to determine the degree and intensity of host response to antigenic challenge, including such assaults as allogeneic tissue transplantation and blood transfusion. The adjective, "allogeneic," when used in this context, denotes the antipathetic relationship that exists between genetically dissimilar members of the same species.

Histocompatibility molecules are serologically detectable. They form cell surface protrusions, yet penetrate to the cell interior, extending a relatively lesser distance from the internal, cytoplasmic surface of the membrane. These integral, but freely mobile, plasma membrane glycoproteins are designated as HLA histocompatibility antigens in Man, and as H-2 antigens in the laboratory mouse (Bach & van Rood, 1976). Histocompatibility specificities characterize white blood cells, platelets, and the surfaces of cells that comprise the fixed tissues of the body, including dendritic Langerhans' cells found within the living layer of the epidermis (Edelson & Fink, 1985).

The molecules of the histocompatibility complex divide into two sub-classes. Some of these molecules (HLA-A, HLA-B, HLA-C) are present on most human body cells as classic transplantation antigens; others (HLA-D, HLA-DR) appear primarily on the outer membranes of B lymphocytes and macrophages. This selective distribution clearly befits molecular structures that can so profoundly influence the recognitive properties of cells.

It is important to point out that there is also a group of genes located within an HLA-D chromosomal subregion that encodes for so-called immune response-associated (Ia) antigens, a class of cell surface marker that has a controlling influence on both immune responsivity and immune suppression (Benacerraf & McDevitt, 1972; Gasser & Silvers, 1984). To know the specificities of this particular gene array has become a priority goal in immunology, in view of the fact that variants ("alleles") of HLA-D gene products have been found to offer reliable markers for the detection of inherited disease susceptibility (Hurley, Giles, & Capra, 1983). The pace at which priorities are being set in the fast-developing field of immunogenetics, then being met forthwith, is demonstrated in a recently achieved milestone: to wit, the characterization and cloning of the major histocompatibility complex itself (Steinmetz & Hood, 1983).

The Influence of MHC Gene Products

Genetic (histocompatibility-linked) control of cellular, T lymphocyte-mediated immunity and humoral, B lymphocyte-mediated immunity can find no better illustration than the manner in which genes of the histocompatibility complex influence the cooperative interaction of the various immune cell subtypes. The fact that descriptions of this interaction should be presented in the literature as a general schematic, subject to change, is testimony to its complexity. We present below two descriptions of cell:cell cooperation involving the regulatory T helper cell, the nonsecretory B lymphocyte and its immunoglobulin (antibody)-secreting plasma cell progeny, and the amoeboid blood monocyte, the macrophage.

T and B cell differentiation and clonal expansion are dependent upon a highly structured process of antigen presentation that is histocompatibility-restricted (Haskins, Kappler, & Marrack, 1984; Meuer et al., 1983; Schwartz, Yano, & Paul, 1978). Lymphocyte activation out of the resting (G_0) phase of the cell cycle is MHC-restricted in the sense that foreign antigen must first be bound by a receptor molecule on the surface of an accessory cell *in association with* a genetically encoded self-antigen (in this case, an Ia gene product). This association may involve the physical interaction of MHC molecule and antigen (Schwartz, 1985).

As accessory cell, the macrophage is thought to process (chemically alter), then present, antigen to the T helper cell in the exact genetically-restricted orientation that will facilitate T cell induction and reactivity (Katz & Benacerraf, 1975; Schwartz, 1984). In turn, the T cell stimulates the B lymphocyte into blastosis and the production of plasma cells and B memory cells (Abney et al., 1978).

In a recent essay, Leserman (1985) has proposed an alternative model of antigen presentation, involving the B lymphocyte, that takes into account biochemical events that precede presentation. Here, the stimulated B cell internalizes antigen in a cross-linkage of surface immunoglobulins, at least one of which forms an association with MHC molecules within the encapsulating vescicle. Then, by means of a mechanism that is "independent of the physical structure of the antigen" (p. 352), partially denatured antibody is reexpressed at the cell surface as part of an *antibody*-MHC complex. In this schematic, antibody, rather then antigen, has become the stimulus to T cell activation, if, and only if, it is complexed to the histocompatibility molecule.

In another illustration of genetic control of immunity, an activated T_4 cell stimulates the B cell through cross linkage, each cell type recognizing a different stereoconfigurative aspect of the immunogen. The resulting "matrix of antigen" no doubt facilitates the binding process, and is also thought to assist memory consolidation in both cell lines (Mitchison, 1971). Once again, it has been found that the salient recognition structures involved are programmed by particular immune response genes (McDevitt et al., 1972).

CONCLUSIONS

One of the more zestful pursuits enjoyed by psychoneuroimmunologists has been their continuing dispute with a central tenet of immunology: the cherished belief (held, they believe, by immunologists at large) that the immune system is a self-governing, self-directing system—that it is in fact autonomous. It is hoped that the point will have been made, in this brief review, that the immune system differs radically from other body systems in certain important respects, and that if it *is* in fact autonomous (which, as we shall see, it is not), its autokinetic properties are not necessarily the source of its uniqueness.

Thus, each of the physiologic systems—neuronal, immune, cardiovascular, and endocrine—is assumed to be strongly integrated by circuits of feedback. Each is understood to be internalized ("autonomous") along dimensions of space and time. In each, in other words, key events at key tissue sites are coordinated, point-to-point, by signal-receptor bonds enchaining complex biophysicochemical sequences and cascades within optimal thresholds. Thus perceived, all physiologic systems are communication systems. It is within this narrow definition of communication, however, that comparison between the immune system and other systems stops.

Hence, in immunologic terms, systems closure is expressed as "network," or "web." The perception, here, is of a *concentric* structure, unique among systems, one that is marked by dynamism, fluidity, and an autonomaticity that holds in balance enormous forces of inhibition (suppression) against an equally enormous potential for self-expansion. Yet, even as it monitors these inner forces in an apparent dialogue of idiotypes, the immune system is assuredly occupied in monitoring the larger circumference, the larger self. The suggestion has been made, it will be recalled, that the system may act as a central monitor for all physiologic systems (Vaz et al., 1984).

With such thoughts in mind, one might suggest (not entirely in jest) that, from their primordial origins, immune molecules and cells have found desirable refuge in legions of obliging hosts, up and down the phyla throughout the eons, their own genetic composition remaining remarkably stable, the while. Survival of this multitudinous host has therefore been paramount, any threat to the individual unit being met with masterfully coordinated, aggressive attack. Excepting that a hospitable environment prevail, the express form and substance of "higher organisms" must be considered utterly incidental. That this substance should incorporate—in one extraordinary instance—an acute and energetic sense of destiny, is without consequence. Such is the philosophy of the true (and successful) parasite.

REFERENCES

Adams, D. O., & Hamilton, T. A. The cell biology of macrophage activation. *Annual Review of Immunology,* 1984, 2, 283-318.
Abney, E. R., Cooper, M. D., Kearney, J. F., Lawton, A. R., & Parkhouse, R. M. Sequential expression of immunoglobulin on developing mouse B lymphocytes: A systematic survey that suggests a model for the generation of immunoglobulin isotype diversity. *Journal of Immunology,* 1978, 120 (6), 2041-2049.

Auerbach, R. Experimental analysis of the origin of cell types in the development of the mouse thymus. *Developmental Biology,* 1961, 3 (3), 336-354.

Bach, J. F., Bach, M. A., Charreire, J., Dardenne, M., & Pleau, J. M. The mode of action of thymic hormones. *Annals of the New York Academy of Sciences,* 1979, 332, 23-32.

Bach, F. H., & van Rood, J. J. The major histocompatibility complex: Genetics and biology (third of three parts). *New England Journal of Medicine,* 1976, 295 (17), 927-936.

Benacerraf, B. Role of MHC gene products in immune regulation. *Science,* 1981, 212 (4500), 1229-1238.

Benacerraf, B., & McDevitt, H. O. Histocompatibility-linked immune response genes. *Science,* 1972, 175 (19), 273-279.

Bhan, A. K., Reinherz, E. L., Poppema, S., McClusky, R. T., & Schlossman, S. F. Location of T cell and major histocompatibility complex antigens in the human thymus. *Journal of Experimental Medicine,* 1980, 152 (4), 771-782.

Billingham, R. E., Brent, L., & Medawar, P. B. 'Actively acquired tolerance' of foreign cells. *Nature (London),* 1953, 172 (4379), 603-606.

Bona, C. A. Regulatory idiotypes. In H. Köhler, J. Urbain, & P. A. Cazenave (Eds.), *Idiotypy in Biology and Medicine.* Orlando: Academic Press, 1984, 29-42.

Bos, J. D., & Kapsenberg, M. L. The skin immune system: Its cellular constituents and their interactions. *Immunology Today,* 1986, 7 (7, 8), 235-240.

Breinl, F., & Haurowitz, F. Chemische Untersuchung des Präzipitates aus Hämoglobin und Anti-Hämoglobin-Serum und Bemerkungen über die Natur der Anti-körper. *Zeitschrift für Physikalischen Chemie, Stochiömetrie und Verwandtschaftslehre,* 1930, 192, 45-57.

Brent, L. The continuing quest for specific unresponsiveness in tissue and organ transplantation. *Cellular Immunology,* 1981, 62 (2), 264-270.

Brent, L., Brooks, C. G., Medawar, P. B., Simpson, E. Transplantation tolerance. *British Medical Bulletin,* 1976, 32 (2), 101-106.

Buckley, R. H. Primary immunodeficiency diseases. In J. B. Wyngaarden, & L. H. Smith (Eds.), *Cecil Textbook of Medicine,* Vol. 2. Philadelphia: W. B. Saunders, 1982, 1789-1796.

Burnet, F. M. *The Clonal Selection Theory of Acquired Immunity.* London: Cambridge University Press, 1959.

Burnet, F. M. Clonal selection and after. In G. I. Bell, A. S. Perelson, & G. H. Pimbley, Jr. (Eds.), *Theoretical Immunology.* New York: Marcel Dekker, 1978, 63-85.

Burnet, F. M., & Fenner, F. *The Production of Antibodies.* 2nd edition. Melbourne: MacMillan, 1949.

Cantor, H., & Boyse, E. A. Functional subclasses of T lymphocytes bearing different Ly antigens. I. The generation of functionally distinct T-cell subclasses is a differentiative process independent of antigen. *Journal of Experimental Medicine,* 1975, 141 (6), 1376-1389.

Claman, H. N., Chaperon, E. A., & Triplett, R. F. Thymus-marrow cell combinations. Synergism in antibody production. *Proceedings of the Society for Experimental Biology and Medicine,* 1966, 122 (4), 1167-1171.

Cohn, M. Why lymphokines? In E. Pick (Ed.), *Lymphokines: A Forum for Immunoregulatory Cell Products. Growth and Differentiation of B Cells,* Vol. 10. New York: Academic Press, 1985, 201-223.

Conley, M. E., Beckwith, J. B., Mancer, J. F., & Tenckhoff, L. The spectrum of the Di George syndrome. *Journal of Pediatrics,* 1979, 94 (6), 883-890.

Cooper, E. L. *General Immunology.* 1st edition. New York: Pergamon Press, 1982.

Dausset, J. Are D and DR two distinct entities? In R. A. Reisfeld, & S. Ferrone (Eds.), *Current Trends in Histocompatibility,* Vol. 1. *Immunogenetic and Molecular Profiles.* New York: Plenum Press, 1981, 29-47.

Deeg, H. J., & Storb, R. Graft-versus-host disease: Pathophysiological and clinical aspects. *Annual Review of Medicine,* 1984, 35, 11-24.

Dorf, M. E., & Benacerraf, B. Suppressor cells and immunoregulation. *Annual Review of Immunology,* 1984, 2, 127-157.

Dumond, D. C., & Hamblin, A. Lymphokines. In E. J. Holborow, & W. G. Reeves (Eds.), *Immunology in Medicine: A Comprehensive Guide to Clinical Immunology.* 2nd edition. New York: Grune & Stratton, 1983, 121-150.

Eardley, D. D., Hugenberger, J., McVay-Boudreau, L., Shen, F. W., Gerson, R. K., & Cantor, H. Immunoregulatory circuits among T-cell sets. I. T-helper cells induce other T-cell sets to exert feedback inhibition. *Journal of Experimental Medicine,* 1978, 147 (4), 1106-1115.

Edelson, R. L., & Fink, J. M. The immunologic function of skin. *Scientific American,* 1985, 252 (6), 46-53.

Erlich, P. The Croonian Lecture. On immunity with special reference to cell life. *Proceedings of the Royal Society (London),* 1900, LXVI (432), 424-448.

Faulk, W. P., & Johnson, P. M. Immunological studies of human placentae: Identification and distribution of proteins in mature chorionic villi. *Clinical and Experimental Immunology,* 1977, 27 (2), 365-375.

Faulk, W. P., & McIntyre, J. A. Trophoblast survival. *Transplantation,* 1981, 32 (1), 1-5.

French, M. E., & Batchelor, J. R. Immunological enhancement of rat kidney grafts. *Lancet,* 1969, 2 (630), 1103-1106.

Gasser, D. I., & Silvers, W. K. Genetic determinants of immunological responsiveness. *Advances in Immunology,* 1974, 18, 1-66.

Goldstein, A. L., & Chirigos, M. A. (Eds.), *Progress in Cancer Research,* Vol. 20. *Lymphokines and Thymic Hormones: Their Potential Utilization in*

Cancer Therapeutics. New York: Raven Press, 1981.

Goldstein, A. L., Thurman, G. B., Low, T. L. K., Rossio, J. L., & Trivers, G. E. Hormonal influences on the reticuloendothelial system: Current status of the role of thymosin in the regulation and modulation of immunity. *Research Journal of the Reticuloendothelial Society,* 1978, 23 (4), 253-266.

Haskins, K., Kappler, J., & Marrack, P. The major histocompatibility complex-restricted antigen receptor on T cells. *Annual Review of Immunology,* 1984, 2, 51-66.

Haurowitz, F. The molecular basis of immunity. *Annals of the New York Academy of Sciences,* 1970, 169 (1), 11-22.

Hauser, S. L., & Weiner, H. L. Cellular regulation of the human immune response and its relation to multiple sclerosis. In P. O. Behan, & F. Spreafico (Eds.), *Neuroimmunology.* (Serono Symposia publications from Raven Press, Vol. 12). New York: Raven Press, 1984, 247-259.

Haynes, B. F. The human thymic microenvironment. *Advances in Immunology,* 1984, 36, 87-142.

Henkart, P. A. Mechanism of lymphocyte-mediated cytotoxicity. *Annual Review of Immunology,* 1985, 3, 31-58.

Hiserodt, J. C., Britvan, L. J., & Targan, S. R. Characterization of the cytolytic reaction mechanism of the human natural killer (NK) lymphocyte: Resolution into binding, programming, and killer cell-independent steps. *Journal of Immunology,* 1982, 129 (4), 1782-1787.

Honjo, T. Immunoglobulin genes. *Annual Review of Immunology,* 1983, 1, 499-528.

Hurley, C. K., Giles, R. C., & Capra, J. D. The human MHC: Evidence for multiple HLA-D-region genes. *Immunology Today,* 1983, 4 (8), 219-226.

Jerne, N. K. Towards a network theory of the immune system. *Annales d'Immunologie (Paris),* 1974, 125C (1-2), 373-389.

Katz, D. H. *Lymphocyte Differentiation, Recognition, and Regulation.* New York: Academic Press, 1977.

Katz, D. H. The immune system: An overview. In D. P. Stites, J. D. Stobo, H. H. Fudenberg, & J. V. Wells (Eds.), *Basic & Clinical Immunology.* 5th edition. Los Altos, California: Lange Medical Publications, 1984, 13-20.

Katz, D. H., & Benacerraf, B. Function and interrelationships of T-cell receptors, Ir genes, and other histocompatibility gene products. *Transplantation Reviews,* 1975, 22, 175-195.

Katz, S. I., Tamaki, K., & Sachs, D. H. Epidermal Langerhans' cells are derived from cells originating in bone marrow. *Nature (London),* 1979, 282 (5736), 324-326.

Kennedy, R. C., Melnick, J. L., & Dreesman, G. R. Anti-idiotypes and immunity. *Scientific American,* 1986, 255 (1), 48-56.

King, A. C., & Cuatrecasas, P. Peptide hormone-induced receptor mobility, aggregation and internalization. *New England Journal of Medicine*, 1981, 305 (2), 77-88.

Kishimoto, T. Factors affecting B cell growth and differentiation. *Annual Review of Immunology*, 1985, 3, 133-157.

Köhler, H. Idiotypic network interactions. *Immunology Today*, 1980, 1, 18-21.

Köhler, H., Levitt, D., & Bach, M. A non-galilean view of the immune network. *Immunology Today*, 1981, 2, 58-60.

Kruisbeek, A. M., Sharrow, S. O., Mathieson, B. J., & Singer, A. The H-2 phenotype of the thymus dictates the self-specificity expressed by thymic but not splenic cytotoxic T lymphocyte precursors in thymus-engrafted mice. *Journal of Immunology*, 1981, 127 (5), 2168-2176.

Kunkel, H. G., Mannick, M., & Williams, R. C. Individual antigenic specificities of isolated antibodies. *Science*, 1963, 140 (3572), 1218-1219.

Lajtha, L. G. Haematopoietic stem cells: Concepts and definitions. *Blood Cells*, 1979, 5 (3), 447-455.

Lane, H. C., & Fauci, A. S. Immunologic abnormalities in the acquired immunodeficiency syndrome. *Annual Review of Immunology*, 1985, 3, 477-500.

Lane, H. C., Depper, J. M., Greene, W. C., Whalen, G., & Waldmann, T. A., & Fauci, A. S. Qualitative analysis of immune function in patients with acquired immunodeficiency syndrome: Evidence for a selective defect in soluble antigen recognition. *New England Journal of Medicine*, 1985, 313 (2), 79-84.

Lane, H. C., Siegel, J. P., Rook, A. H., Masur, H., Gelmann, E. P., Quinnan, G. V., & Fauci, A. S. Use of interleukin-2 in patients with acquired immunodeficiency syndrome. *Journal of Biological Response Modifiers*, 1984, 3 (5), 512-516.

Leserman, L. The introversion of the immune response: A hypothesis for T-B interaction. *Immunology Today*, 1985, 6 (12), 352-355.

Leslie, R. G. Q., & Cohen, S. The active sites of immunoglobulin molecules. In I. Roitt (Ed.), *Essays in Fundamental Immunology: 1*. London: Blackwell Scientific Publications, 1973, 1-27.

Manser, T., Wysocki, L. J., Gridley, T., Near, R. I., & Gefter, M. L. The molecular evolution of the immune response. *Immunology Today*, 1985, 6 (3), 94-101.

Marchalonis, J. J. Surface immunoglobulins of B and T lymphocytes: Molecular properties, association with the cell membrane, and a unified model of antigen recognition. *Contemporary Topics in Molecular Immunology*, 1976, 5, 125-160.

McDevitt, H. L., Deak, B. D., Schreffler, D. C., Klein, J., Stimpfling, J. H., & Snell, G. D. Genetic control of the immune response: Mapping of the Ir-1 locus. *Journal of Experimental Medicine*, 1972, 135(6), 1259-1278.

McFarlin, D. E. Immunological abnormalities associated with neurological diseases. In P. O. Behan, & F. Spreafico (Eds.), *Neuroimmunology*. (Serono Symposia publications from Raven Press, Vol. 12). New York: Raven Press, 1984, 237-245.

Meuer, S. C., Cooper, D. A., Hodgdon, J. C., Hussey, R. E., Fitzgerald, K. A., Schlossman, S. F., & Reinherz, E. L. Identification of the receptor for antigen and major histocompatibility complex on human inducer T lymphocytes. *Science*, 1983, 222 (4629), 1239-1242.

Miller, J. F. A. P. Effect of thymectomy on the immunological responsiveness of the mouse. *Proceedings of the Royal Society of London.* (Series B)., 1962, 156, 415-428.

Mitchison, N. A. The carrier effect in the secondary response to hapten-protein conjugates. II. Cellular cooperation. *European Journal of Immunology*, 1971, 1(2), 18-27.

Morimoto, C., Reinherz, E. L., Abe, T., Homma, M., & Schlossman, S. F. Characteristics of anti-T cell antibodies in systemic lupus erythematosus: Evidence for selective reactivity with normal suppressor cells defined by monoclonal antibodies. *Clinical Immunology and Immunopathology*, 1980, 16 (4), 474-484.

Nathan, C. F., & Cohn, Z. A. Cellular components of inflammation: Monocytes and macrophages. In W. Kelly, E. Harris, S. Ruddy, & C. B. Sledge (Eds.), *Textbook of Rheumatology*. 2nd edition, Vol. I. Philadelphia: W. B. Saunders, 1985, 144-169.

Nossal, G. J. V. Cellular mechanisms of immunological tolerance. *Annual Review of Immunology*, 1983, 1, 33-62.

Nossal, G. J. V., & Pike, B. L. Antibody receptor diversity and diversity of signals. In M. Fougereau & J. Dausset (Eds.), *International Congress of Immunology (4th: 1980: Paris). Immunology 80. Progress in Immunology IV*. New York: Academic Press, 1980, 136-152.

Oldham, R. K. Biological Response Modifiers Programme and cancer chemotherapy. *International Journal of Tissue Reactions*, 1982, 4 (3), 173-188.

O'Sullivan, M. J., McIntyre, J. A., Prior, M., Warriner, G., & Faulk, W. P. Identification of human trophoblast membrane antigens in maternal blood during pregnancy. *Clinical and Experimental Immunology*, 1982, 48 (1), 279-287.

Oudin, J., & Casenave, P. A. Similar idiotypic specificities in immunoglobulin fractions with different antibody functions or even without detectable antibody function. *Proceedings of the National Academy of Sciences, U.S.A.*, 1971, 68 (10), 2616-2620.

Oudin, J., & Michel, M. Une nouvelle forme d'allotypie des globulines gamma du sérum de lapin, apparement liée à la fonction et à la specificité anticorps.

Comptes Rendues de l'Academie de Sciences, 1963, 257 (3), 805-808.

Owen, R. D. Immunogenetic consequences of vascular anastomoses between bovine twins. *Science,* 1945, 102 (2651), 400-401.

Pahwa, R. N., Pahwa, S. G., & Good, R. A. T lymphocyte differentiation in severe combined immunodeficiency defects of the thymus. *Clinical Immunology and Immunopathology,* 1978, 11, 437-444.

Pastan, I. H., & Willingham, M. C. Journey to the center of the cell: Role of the receptosome. *Science,* 1981, 214 (4520), 504-509.

Pick, E. (Ed.), *Lymphokines: A Forum for Immunoregulatory Cell Products.* New York: Academic Press, 1984.

Plaut, M., Bubbers, J. E., & Henney, C. S. Studies of the mechanism of lymphocyte-mediated cytolysis. VII. Two stages in the T cell-mediated lytic cycle with distinct cation requirements. *Journal of Immunology,* 1976, 116 (1), 150-155.

Reinherz, E. L., & Schlossman, S. F. The differentiation and function of human T lymphocytes. *Cell,* 1980, 19 (4), 821-827.

Rocklin, R. E., Bendtzen, K., & Greineder, D. Mediators of immunity: Lymphokines and monokines. *Advances in Immunology,* 1980, 29, 56-136.

Rocklin, R. E., Kitzmiller, J. L., Carpenter, C. B., Garovoy, M. R., & David, J. R. Maternal-fetal relation: Absence of an immunologic blocking factor from the serum of women with chronic abortions. *New England Journal of Medicine,* 1976, 295 (22), 1209-1213.

Schwartz, R. H. The role of gene products of the major histocompatibility complex in T cell activation and cellular interactions. In W. E. Paul (Ed.), *Fundamental Immunology.* New York: Raven Press, 1984, 379-438.

Schwartz, R. H. T-lymphocyte recognition of antigen in association with gene products of the major histocompatibility complex. *Annual Review of Immunology,* 1985, 3, 237-261.

Schwartz, R. H., Yano, A., & Paul, W. E. Interaction between antigen-presenting cells and primed T lymphocytes: An assessment of Ir gene expression in the antigen-presenting cell. *Immunology Reviews,* 1978, 40, 153-180.

Smith, K. Inside the thymus. *Immunology Today,* 1984, 5 (4), 83-84.

Steinmetz, M., & Hood, L. Genes of the major histocompatibility complex in mouse and man. *Science,* 1983, 222 (4625), 440-443.

Stobo, J. D. Lymphocytes. I. T cells. In D. P. Stites, J. D. Stobo, H. H. Fudenberg, & J. V. Wells (Eds.), *Basic & Clinical Immunology.* 5th edition. Los Altos, California: Lange Medical Publications, 1984, 69-76.

Strober, S. Natural suppressor (NS) cells, neonatal tolerance, and total lymphoid irradiation: Exploring obscure relationships. *Annual Review of Immunology,* 1984, 2, 219-237.

Thomas, L. *The Lives of a Cell: Notes of a Biology Watcher.* New York: Viking Press, 1974.

Theofilopoulos, A. N. Autoimmunity. In D. P. Stites, J. D. Stobo, H. H. Fudenberg, J. V. Wells (Eds.), *Basic & Clinical Immunology.* 5th edition. Los Altos, California: Lange Medical Publications, 1984, 152-186.

Vaz, N. M., Martinez-A. C., & Coutinho, A. The uniqueness and boundaries of the idiotypic self. In H. Köhler, J. Urbain, & P. A. Cazenave (Eds.), *Idiotypy in Biology and Medicine.* New York: Academic Press, 1984, 43-59.

Wall, R., & Kuehl, M. Biosynthesis and regulation of immunoglobulins. *Annual Review of Immunology,* 1983, 1, 393-422.

Wilkinson, P. C. Mononuclear phagocytes and granulocytes. In E. J. Holborow, & W. G. Reeves (Eds.), *Immunology in Medicine: A Comprehensive Guide to Clinical Immunology.* 2nd edition. New York: Grune & Stratton, 1983, 60-78.

BIBLIOGRAPHY

Bellanti, J. A. *Immunology III.* Philadelphia: W. B. Saunders Company, 1985.

Bier, O., da Silva, W. D., Gotze, D., & Mota, I. *Fundamentals of Immunology.* New York: Springer Verlag, 1981.

Conn, P. M. (Ed.), *The Receptors,* Vol. 1. Orlando: Academic Press, 1984.

Eisen, H. N. *Immunology: An Introduction to Molecular and Cellular Principles of the Immune Responses.* 2nd edition. Hagerstown, Maryland: Harper & Row, Publishers, 1981.

Holborow, E. J., & W. G. Reeves (Eds.), *Immunology in Medicine: A Comprehensive Guide to Clinical Immunology.* New York: Grune & Stratton, 1983.

Köhler, H., Urbain, J., & Cazenave, P. A. (Eds.), *Idiotypy in Biology and Medicine.* Orlando: Academic Press, 1984.

Pick, E. (Ed.), *Lymphokines: A Forum for Immunoregulatory Products,* Vol 9. New York: Academic Press, 1984.

Schreier, M. H., & K. A. Smith (Eds.), *Lymphokines: Growth and Differentiation of B Cells,* Vol. 10. New York: Academic Press, 1985.

Silverstein, A. M. History of immunology. Development of the concept of immunologic specificity, I. *Cellular Immunology,* 1982, 67 (2), 396-409.

Stites, D. P., Stobo, J. D., Fudenberg, H. H., & Wells, J. V. (Eds.), *Basic & Clinical Immunology.* Los Altos, California: Lange Medical Publications, 1984.

Zinkernagel, R. M., & Doherty, P. C. MHC-restricted cytotoxic T cells: Studies on the biologic role of polymorphic major transplantation antigens determining T cell restriction-specificity, function, and responsiveness. *Advances in Immunology,* 1979, 27, 51-177.

Chapter 3

The Interaction of Systems

The phrase "interaction of systems" has a double meaning. It can mean communication between systems or it may solely convey the idea of influence and counter influence. Nervous, endocrine, and immune systems differ with respect to the kinds of stimulus induction to which each responds. This being so, can true communication take place between them? Communication implies a common language. Is such commonality possible when dimensions of response within any one system must necessarily fall within the constraints of physicochemical imperatives unique to that system—unique both to its complement of signal molecules and to its target structures?

There is evidence to justify the view that the term *interaction*, when used in this present sense, in fact conveys both meanings. It is by now well known that the brain and pituitary gland influence the activity of the endocrine system through complicated neural and neurosecretory pathways, and that the brain itself is a target for endocrine influence. As we shall see, the central nervous system exercises a modulating influence on the immune system. Were the axis of influence to be reversed, we would find that thymus gland hormones, as well as secretions from activated lymphoid cells, feed back upon the brain in ways that can influence both endocrine and immune responsivity.

Should phasic effects taking place within a single system be reflected in related effects, reciprocal or otherwise, within one or both of the other two systems, one might then assume that "information channels"—channels of true communication—were in operation between them (Besedovsky, del Rey, & Sorkin, 1985a). It could be further assumed that such channels were made viable by like codes of communication.

It might still be reasonable to ask *why* such codes should exist. After all, each of the three systems behaves as an independent unit programmed to meet the basal metabolic requirements of particular groupings of organs and cells, unique in type and number. What biological requirement might each have for the other, and to what selective advantage must the three act in consort (Mayr, 1978)? To what extent is the tonic activity of the endocrine system dependent upon input from nerve nets and circulating lymphocytes? Seen from the opposite vantage point, to what extent is brain homeostasis dependent upon the backflow of "tropic" hormones and glucocorticoids along the infundibular corridor? What effect upon brain has the infiltration of thymic peptides? Do the latter also reside in situ? and if so, why? To what degree might the endocrine activity of thymus gland, or lymphocyte, be dependent upon steroid influence? Or, to carry the obvious circularity of all this back to starting point: to what possible purpose do lymphocytes produce pituitary hormone-like molecules, if not to contribute to the regulatory axis controlling the adrenal gland?

At a time when the accelerated pace of discovery—spurred on by the monoclonal probe—is dismantling the traditional view of systems, blurring textbook definitions, and generally stirring up knotty problems of classification and semantics, these are questions to ponder. Furthermore, there is already a wealth of evidence, chiefly resulting from the intensive study of brain peptides, to indicate that a given "classical" neurotransmitter can behave as neurohormone, a neurohormone as neurotransmitter, and either as neuromodulator (Siggins, 1978), depending upon such factors as the intrinsic spontaneous activity and environmental matrix of the effector cell, the locus, speed, and duration of its biological action, and the stable and dynamic characteristics of receptor sites (Barchas et al., 1978; Rotsztejn, 1980). It is also known that "a particular peptide may exercise different effects at different sites by different mechanisms, doubtless in response to different stimuli" (Defendini & Zimmerman, 1978, p. 138).

When the potential neuroendocrine modulatory capacity of the immune system is introduced into the picture, as recent research reports ostensibly warrant, it becomes something of an understatement to describe the data base for psychoneuroimmunology as "complicated." In view of these complications, this chapter will begin with a broad sketch of the patterns of interaction suggested by these data, only later listing specific details.

First of all, however, an introduction to some central players in these convoluted processes is in order.

From the biochemical point of view, the story of immune-neuroendocrine interrelationships is essentially a story of peptides. The patterns of interaction in question are therefore familial in character, common properties bestowing upon kindred substances the resemblance expected of family members. Indeed, in view of the striking homology found among peptides belonging, in the classical sense, to different systems, it becomes impossible to ignore certain intriguing implications for psychoneuroimmunology that derive from these similarities, as well as impossible not to suggest still other parallels worthy of investigation.

It would of course be correct to surmise that peptidergic cells—given their structural and chemical homology—must share a common ancestry, whatever their ultimate tissue distribution in adult organisms. The secretory cell systems of the brain and pituitary that are the source of peptide "releasing" and "tropic" hormones governing neuroendocrine and endocrine activity are derivatives of the neural crest, neuroectoderm, and ectoblast (Said, 1980). The peptide-producing cells of the gut also originate from the neural crest (Pictet et al., 1976), as does the thymus gland (Cooper, 1982). By way of illustration, Bockman and Kirby (1985) have shown that normal development of the thymus is either prevented, or seriously compromised, by ablation of small portions of embryonic neural crest tissue.

Bioactive peptides are actually molecular fragments. In contrast to the enzymatically controlled synthesis of conventional neurotransmitters from amino acids and monoamines, the peptide hormones are synthesized on RNA template within the cell nucleus by proteolytic conversion of a genetically-encoded, macromolecular glycoprotein (Docherty & Steiner, 1982; Eipper & Mains, 1980). The fragmentation by enzymatic transformation of the parent peptide molecule is a highly selective and subtle determinant of peptide function, as well as an important aspect of peptide synthesis. Different fragments of the same peptide, differing, in some instances, by no more than a single amino acid, can differ as much in their functional properties as do different peptides of the same general class.

The opiomelanocortins, ACTH and beta-endorphin, provide a striking example of this characteristic. Differentially processed from the same glycoprotein, pro-opiomelanocortin (POMC), the two peptides are localized within the same nerve cells bodies, occupy the same pituitary cells, and are released stoichiometrically from the same secretory granules (Agnati et al., 1982; Guillemin et al., 1977). Yet, ACTH and β-endorphin differ in their behavioral effects, not alone from one another, but intrinsically as well, particular amino acid fragments of a single peptide molecule apparently reflecting, in each case, unique receptor affinities (Bohus, 1984).

Peptides are ubiquitous. A peptide might first be discovered in the brain, only to be subsequently isolated from intestinal tissue, pancreas, or lung. The converse is as likely to be true. The polypeptide gastrointestinal hormone, cholecystokinin (CCK), originally found in the duodenal and jejunal mucosa (Rayford, Miller, & Thompson, 1976a, 1976b), has lately been isolated from brain tissue (Beinfeld et al., 1983; Gaudreau et al., 1985). Or, to cite a second such example, the "richest source" of the anomalous, nonsecretory "thymic" peptide, thymosin β_4, is not the thymus gland, but the spleen—the thymus, the respiratory epithelium, and the brain comprising three, among several, secondary sources for the hormone (Horecker & Morgan, 1984).

HORMONES AND THE BRAIN; A NEURO-ENDOCRINE-LYMPHOID AXIS?

The pituitary gland, i.e., *hypophysis* (Gr., undergrowth), enjoys its reputation as the master endocrine gland of the body in part because of its strategic position. From the brain itself, the gland receives indirect stimulation from afferent fiber networks that converge on the medial hypothalamus from the neocortex, thalamus, limbic structures, preoptic area, midbrain, and brainstem (Anschel, Alexander, & Perachio, 1982; Renaud, Pittman, & Blume, 1979; Zaborsky, 1982).

Collaterals from each of these networks also innervate the median eminence (infundibulum), a unique hypothalamic tissue situated immediately superior to the pituitary gland. Described as a "pulsatile system," the median eminence is a small, interstitial space in which enzymes, transmitters, and neurohormones mingle in high concentration (Joseph & Knigge, 1978; Kobayashi, Matsui, & Ishii, 1970; Kordon et al., 1979). Not surprisingly, the structure is recognized as neurohemal end-organ for the entire hypothalamic-hypophysiotropic complex. It may be surmised that it is crucial to the integration of nervous, neuroendocrine, endocrine, and immune systems (see Lloyd, 1984, for review).

In short, the hypothalamic-hypophysial region of the brain is acknowledged to be *the* primary site for the biological transformation (transduction) of sensory input received both from without and within the organism. Here, brain-endocrine interaction evidently takes place along a glial-vascular chain (Löfgren, 1959a, 1959b), a meshwork of anastomotic arteries and fenestrated capillaries fostering a diversified pattern of flow within the pituitary gland itself, as well as between it, the carotid arterial circulation, the third ventricle of the brain, and the cerebrospinal fluid (Bergland & Page, 1979).

The fine structure and pharmacology of the central neurons and neurosecretory cells whose fibers intersect this area are being defined, with ever more clarity, by dramatic advances in exploratory techniques. Having made possible the complete characterization of brain transmitter systems, this technology is also bringing to light previously unsuspected varieties of anatomical, bioelectric, and biochemical relationship between and within cell groups.

This prodigious research effort is reflected in an extensive literature. Rather than digress from our central theme to review what has been more appropriately summarized elsewhere (Lloyd, 1984; Zaborszky, 1982), we will focus on the ways in which the immune system influences, and is in turn influenced by, other important regulatory circuits. Beyond doubt, brain chemistry, the activated components of the immune system, and the secretory products of endocrine glands form a labyrinthian network. It will be our purpose, in this present chapter, to show where and how their interaction takes place, as well as to address the more interesting question: why?

Equilibria Among Systems

The pituitary gland is the source of tropic endocrine hormones that control the activity of the other endocrine glands of the body: namely, the adrenals, the thyroid, and the reproductive organs. In addition, it is now known that hormones whose central influence was once presumed limited to the dynamics of their own release, i.e., to the negative feedback inhibition of their hypophysial "releasing" factors, enter the brain, and that they may do so at varying rates, and by more than one route (Bergland et al., 1980; Dunn & Gispen, 1977; Jones et al., 1982).

Studied extensively over the past 30 years, the hypothalamic-pituitary-adrenal axis offers a classic model of inhibitory feedback in physiologic systems. The secretion of corticotropin-releasing hormone (CRH) (corticoliberin) from the paraventricular nucleus of the hypothalamus is modulated by the long-loop feedback of its peripheral products, i.e., the anterior pituitary tropic hormone, corticotropin (ACTH), and the adrenal steroids, cortisol and corticosterone (de Kloet, Veldhuis, & Bohus, 1980; Vale et al., 1984).

The "opposite and competing influences" of the releasing hormone, corticoliberin, and the peripheral tissue steroids evidently control ACTH release at the most fundamental level. As antagonists, they have been shown to modulate the rate of transcription of the ACTH precursor molecule gene, i.e., the gene controlling production of the prohormone, pro-opiomelanocortin (POMC),[*] as well as the rate of peptide release (Gagner & Drouin, 1985).

In sum, bidirectionality is an essential feature of a control system whose mode of operation is otherwise relatively straightforward. That is to say, despite its signal property of feedback, the system has been perceived as centrally controlled, as hierarchical; or, to perceive it geometrically, as pyramidal in structure. Now, however, in the face of new evidence on immune and neuroendocrine interaction, a shift in perspective has changed the vantage point, and we find ourselves attempting to understand a tangle of interconnections and interdependencies whose significance is far from clear. The balance of these introductory remarks will include a synopsis of these recent experimental findings, as well as a cautious interpretation of data published, to date, in a small and relatively select literature.

In the most general terms, it can be stated that hormonal substances produced and released by the immune system may be affected by some of the same control vectors as those that govern the output of the endocrine glands. The more significant point to emphasize, however, is that immune components have not only been shown to be sensitive to these controls, but to contribute to them—to show themselves capable, in other words, of regulating the regulators.

To illustrate: soluble products of the immune system, such as thymic hormones and lymphokines, are thought to enter the brain to effectuate the synthesis and release of the monoamine neurotransmitter, norepinephrine (Besedovsky et al., 1983). Norepinephrine, in turn, inhibits the synthesis and release of still other neurotransmitter substances (serotonin, acetylcholine) capable of stimulating the output of the hypothalamic releasing hormone, corticoliberin (Jones, Hillhouse, & Burden, 1976). Immunologic stimulus to this primary inhibitory action by norepinephrine of course prevents corticoliberin from activating the hypophysial-adrenal axis.

This interaction makes perfect biological sense, so far. Here, as we can see, is a counterbalance: the inhibition of corticoliberin prevents elevated levels of circulating glucocorticoids from selectively suppressing an early,

---

[*]Adrenocorticotropin, or ACTH, melanocyte-stimulating hormone (MSH), methionine [Met]-enkephalin, and the biologically inactive pro-hormone of the endorphins, β-lipotropin (β-LPH), have all been found to be synthesized *de novo* from pro-opiomelanocortin (POMC), a macromolecular glycoprotein found in endocrine cells in the anterior hypophysis (Chrétien et al., 1979; Cohen et al., 1980; Eipper & Mains, 1978; Mains, Eipper, & Ling, 1977; Roberts & Herbert, 1977a, 1977b), as well as in nerve cell bodies in the arcuate nucleus of the hypothalamus (Liotta et al., 1979; Pelletier, 1980).

critical phase of the immune response (Besedovsky & Sorkin, 1977; Hall et al., 1985b).

Regrettably, the varieties of modulatory effects impinging on steroid production hardly allow for orderly arrangement and interpretation. Two additional examples suffice to make the point: hormone-like substances released by peripheral lymphocytes (lymphokines) and monocytes (monokines) are capable of *enhancing* steroidogenesis!—this enhancement presumably preventing the clonal expansion of lymphocytes and accessory cells with low affinity for antigen (Besedovsky et al., 1985a). Then too, a "new regulatory pathway" in the maze is indicated by the finding that a product of lipopolysaccharide (LPS)-treated peritoneal, and bone marrow-derived, murine macrophages can exercise a direct, pronounced, and persistent *suppression* of steroidogenesis in explanted rabbit adrenocortical cells (Mathison et al., 1983).

These bewildering, seemingly contradictory data have been reviewed by two leading investigative teams currently at work in this difficult research area (Besedovsky et al., 1985a; Hall et al., 1985a, 1985b). Assembling present evidence, they argue the following: (1) Peptide hormones of the thymus gland fulfill an important regulatory role in the hypothalamic-hypophysial-adrenal feedback circuit. (2) In performing this role, thymic products impact directly on the brain itself, only indirectly influencing the pituitary and adrenal glands. (3) These same hormones may be endogenous to particular areas of the central nervous system. (4) Thymic factors, such as thymosin fraction 5 (TSN-5) and facteur thymique serique (FTS), most probably "down-regulate" glucocorticoid receptors on circulating lymphocytes—still another "opposite and competing" influence—rendering the cells less susceptible to elevated serum steroid levels. (5) The presence of these same factors in brain may also act to "disinhibit" the inhibitory effect of steroid feedback on central tissues. (6) Finally, "the possibility of synergism" (Hall et al., 1985a) between peptide hormones of the thymus gland and the hypothalamic releasing hormone, corticoliberin, is real, and obviously presents an investigative challenge of some significance. As we shall see, a like relationship to corticoliberin has now been established for the antidiuretic hormone and neurosecretory product of the posterior hypothalamus, vasopressin[*] (Brownstein, Russell, & Gainer, 1980), which, like corticoliberin, is synthesized in the arcuate paraventricular nucleus (Bloom et al., 1982; Cummings et al., 1983).

---

[*]Vasopressin, corticoliberin, and two fragments of the dynorphin molecule, dynorphin-A-(1-8) and dynorphin-A-(1-17), all originate in hypothalamic magnocellular nuclei (Goldstein & Ghazarossian, 1980), whence they enter the posterior pituitary secretory pathway.

If such a relationship between brain and thymus were to be confirmed through future experiment, it would be difficult not to acknowledge that autoregulatory centers for neuroendocrine and immune integration are dispersed, rather than wholly centralized; that axes (if that term should remain appropriate) are *multi-*, not solely *bi*directional; that reciprocal effects are legion, and are themselves sensitive to reversals of "field;" that systems, understood in the conventional sense to be closed, are in fact open and penetrable by other systems; and, finally, that properties such as these latter might more appropriately be said to characterize a "suprasystem," a complex overlay of subsystems operating in continuous flux as an enormous, yet *single* regulatory unit. Were we to return, at this point, to our geometric simile, we might well find our pyramid transformed, and in its place, an interlocking series of greater and lesser spheres.

A Neuroendocrine Role for Thymic Hormones: Preliminary Evidence

There now exists a sizable body of research showing anatomic and functional connection between the brain and the tissues of immunity. Points of possible intersection have been a primary area of interest in the field of neuroimmunomodulation, a research specialty grounded in the investigative techniques of neuro- and immunophysiology (see Spector & Korneva, 1981; Spector, 1986; Stein, Schleifer, & Keller, 1981, for reviews). Whereas its general findings are not of direct relevance to the topic of this present section, there are particular findings that can help to provide a background, and are relevant, as well, to a later discussion of modulatory effects between systems.

For example, a direct preganglionic cholinergic pathway has been found to connect brainstem nuclei, spinal cord neurons, and the thymus gland (Bulloch & Moore, 1981). Autonomic innervation of the thymus, lymph nodes, and spleen has also been amply documented (Crotti, 1918; Fujiwara, Muryobayashi, & Shimamoto, 1966; Giron, Crutcher, & Davis, 1980; Hammar, 1935; Reilly et al., 1979; Williams et al., 1981). In addition, the immunomodulatory role of the central nervous system is clearly evident in the changes brought about in various parameters of immunologic integrity and function (e.g., thymic size, lymphocyte blastogenesis, adherent spleen cell activity, anaphylactic response, etc.) by electrolytic lesioning of the amygdala and hippocampus (immune enhancement) (Roszman et al., 1982), as well as lesioning, ablation, and stimulation of the anterior hypothalamus (immunosuppression) (Cross et al., 1980; Roszmann et al., 1985; Spector & Korneva, 1981; Stein et al., 1981).

An *afferent* pathway between peripheral sites of acute inflammatory response and the brain has been demonstrated in the work of Hugo Besedovsky and colleagues. They have shown that individual neurons in the ventromedial nucleus of the hypothalamus in preimmunized rats increase in firing frequency following systemic administration of antigen (sheep red blood cells [SRBC] or trinitrophenylated-hemacyanin [TNP-Hae]) (Besedovsky et al., 1977). A later study by this same group describes a marked decrease in norepinephrine synthesis (turnover rate) in the hypothalamus of the rat, following the systemic injection of either SRBC or supernatant derived from concanavalin A-stimulated lymphoid cells (Besedovksy et al., 1983).

Thymic Hormone as "Releasing Hormone"

Several interesting findings point to a neuroendocrine role for peptide hormones produced by the thymus gland. Evidence collected to date strongly implies their regulatory feedback to the central nervous system. Given its recency, this evidence is somewhat fragmentary. Consequently, any listing of the more important of these findings must lack cohesion, save that the thymus unquestionably emerges as an integral participant in brain-endocrine interaction.

One: extensive thymosin alpha$_1$-like immunoreactivity (Goldstein et al., 1977; Low et al., 1979; Palaszynski et al., 1983) has been demonstrated in rat brain tissue, with highest concentrations detected in the tuberal region of the hypothalamus, i.e., the arcuate nucleus, ventromedial nucleus, and median eminence (Hall et al., 1982; Palaszynski et al., 1983). Two: the thymus extract, thymosin fraction 5 (TSN-F5), will increase adrenal weight in adult male rats, when injected via chronic implant into these same areas (Hall et al., 1985b). Three: this same heterogeneous extract of thymus peptides exhibits corticoliberin-like activity when administered by femoral cannulation to "unanesthetized, freely moving, undisturbed" premenarcheal primates (cynomolgus monkeys, *Macaca fascicularis*). The peptide brings about increased levels in plasma of ACTH, cortisol, and the opiate peptide, beta-endorphin (Healy et al., 1983). Moreover, it has been seen that TSN-F5 elicits a time- and dose-dependent increase in serum corticosterone when injected intraperitoneally in rodents (McGillis et al., 1985). Four: consistent with the above findings is the discovery that a 43-amino acid component of TSH-F5, thymosin beta$_4$ (TSN-β_4), will elicit the release of luteinizing hormone-releasing hormone (LHRH) from medial basal hypothalamic tissue, and from pituitary tissue superfused with hypothalamic tissue, *in vitro* (Rebar et al., 1981). The intraventricular injection of this same hormone, TSN-β_4, will cause a significant increase in serum luteinizing hormone (LH) levels in chronically cannulated mice (Hall et al., 1982).

Healy et al. (1983) have proposed that the corticotropin (ACTH)-releasing activity of the thymus might reside "in a vasopressin-like amino acid sequence that is either normally present in this gland, or is a derivative of some larger thymic peptide" (p. 1355). Granted that the thymic factor is unknown at the present time, as are the mechanisms that would explain these provocative findings, these investigators nevertheless offer two suggestions: (1) the thymus might *itself* produce a neurohormone- or corticoliberin (CRH)-like substance capable of initiating the enzymatic conversion of pro-opiomelanocortin, the parent molecule for ACTH, the endorphin family, and the enkephalins; or (2), the mechanism might be indirect and synergic, the putative polypeptide entering the brain to stimulate the release of *hypothalamic* CRH.

These speculations by Healy and his group are not far from the mark. Vincent Geenen and coworkers in Liège have reported the presence of the nonapeptide hormone, oxytocin, and its carrier protein, neurophysin, in the human thymus. This discovery indicates that either thymocytes, or stromal cells of the thymic matrix, produce hormones identical to those produced by the magnocellular neurosecretory system of the hypothalamus (Geenen et al., 1986).

What is a Lymphokine?

Lymphocytes and cells of the mononuclear phagocytic system (i.e., monocytes, macrophages) produce a group of peptides that are similar, if not identical, in function and structure to the peptide products of neurosecretory cells. Needless to say, a number of interesting hypotheses are being entertained as a result of this discovery.

To begin, there is compelling evidence at hand that the immune system may serve in a "sensory" capacity, receiving through the channels of the lymphatic system, and transmitting to the brain, information essential to the inviolability of the host (Blalock, 1984a). It becomes increasingly apparent that this faculty depends upon a set of signal molecules and receptors common to both the immune and neuroendocrine systems, and that the two systems may be joined together through a wholly integrated, reciprocal circuitry (Blalock, 1984a, 1984b; Smith, Johnson, & Blalock, 1984).

Present writings that attempt to interpret the new knowledge of lymphokines, monokines, and thymosin peptides reveal the strain imposed on the writer by the encumbrances of a nomenclature that is specific to sys-

tems. The search for appropriate descriptors has become an on-going af-
fair. As a case in point, the term "immunotransmitter" has been recently introduced to convey the range of effects on body cells, including nerve
cells, induced by these groups of proteins (Hall et al., 1985a). Nor are the
semantic discriminations that are the essential yardstick for accurate definition in biology likely to become easier with time. As J. Edwin Blalock
has observed: "in the future, it may be difficult to distinguish the receptors
and signals that these systems use for communication within and between
one another" (p. 1067). He makes the additional point that peptide *function* may prove no less ambiguous a marker: if immunoregulatory
cytokines can behave as neuroendocrines, should it seem remarkable that
hormones produced by the brain and pituitary fulfill an immunoregulatory
role (Blalock, 1984a)?

How Universal a Language?

A diligent search for receptor specificity in lymphoid tissues has offered
incontrovertible evidence that the thymus, spleen, and individual immune
cells offer binding sites to numerous bioactive ligands produced from nervous and neuroendocrine tissue. A partial list of those ligands found on the
membrane surfaces of lymphocytes would include vasoactive intestinal
peptide (VIP) (Danek et al., 1983), β-endorphin (Hazum, Chang, &
Cuatrecasas, 1979), acetylcholine (Maśliński, Grabczewaska, & Ryzewski,
1980), substance P (Payan, Brewster, & Goetzl, 1984), somatostatin
(Bhathena et al., 1981), insulin (Gavin et al., 1973), norepinephrine
(Pochet et al., 1979), dopamine (Stepién et al., 1981), and enkephalin
(Wybran et al., 1979). In addition, immunocytochemical observation has
shown cholecystokinin (CCK)-like and Met-enkephalin-like immune
reactivity in the spleen, as well as VIP-like immunoreactivity in the cortex
of the thymus gland (Felten et al., 1985).

The conviction grows that circulating white blood cells must act as one
locus of origin, among many, for the transmittal of peripheral information
to the brain. Precisely how their "sensory" messages are so conveyed
remains unclear, yet new data have made it tempting to believe that the
molecular signals emanating from peripheral leukocytes (these signals already known to act as neuromodulators) may ultimately be found to include neurotransmitters or related molecules (Blalock, 1984b). Certainly,
it is not now considered beyond the realm of possibility that, depending
upon immune cell type and chosen stimulus, "...the immune system may
produce many if not all of the known neuroendocrine peptide hormones"
(Blalock, Harbour-McMenamin, & Smith, 1985, p. 858s).

If evidence to support this contention is not yet cohesive, it is nevertheless impressive. The following observations suggest the possible extent of immune system input to axes of hormonal control:

Steroid hormone production by the adrenal cortex is significantly reduced in mice treated from birth with rabbit antibody to mouse immunoglobulin M (IgM) mu-chain and subsequently exposed to herpes simplex virus infection of the eye. In other words, a negligible rise in corticosteroid levels is seen in virus-infected, selectively immunosuppressed (i.e., B lymphocyte-depleted) mice, as compared to a marked rise in steroid level noted in control animals (Jordan et al., as reported in Blalock & Smith, 1985).

With respect to the cellular branch of the immune system, T lymphocytes produce endorphins (Smith & Blalock, 1981) and, when exposed to the bacterial toxin, *Staphylococcus* enterotoxin A, synthesize the endocrine hormone, thyrotropin, in culture (Smith et al., 1983). The T cell lymphokine, interferon (IFN), a peptide that is antigenically and structurally similar to ACTH (Smith, Meyer, & Blalock, 1982), acts as a corticotropin-like stimulus to adrenal cells, *in vitro* (Blalock & Harp, 1981; Chany et al., 1980). Corroborative data, derived *in vivo*, have shown the injection of lymphokine-containing supernatant, obtained from mitogen-activated rat spleen cells and human peripheral blood leukocytes, to cause a two- to three-fold increase in circulating corticosterone levels in the rat (Besedovsky, del Rey, & Sorkin, 1981).

Data on active substances derived from monocytes, again validated by observations in laboratory animals judged against the results of cell culture, have shown: (1) the cloned murine monokine, interleukin 1 (rIl-1), and a combination of the neuropeptides, corticoliberin and arginine vasopressin, are equipotent in eliciting ACTH release from mouse pituitary tumor cells (AtT-20), *in vitro* (Woloski et al., 1985); and (2) the intraperitoneal injection in normal and athymic mice of either natural interleukin 1 (Il-1), or the recombinant form of the monokine, stimulates a "severalfold" increase in blood levels of ACTH and corticosterone (Besedovsky et al., 1986). Whether this particular cytokine activates the pituitary-adrenal axis at the level of the pituitary gland (by stimulating ACTH secretion), or at the level of the hypothalamus (by stimulating the secretion of corticoliberin), is a question this most recent study leaves unanswered.

The extension of this idea, namely, that peptides produced by the immune system might altogether by-pass the hypothalamic-pituitary axis to *directly* stimulate steroid production, has been successfully put to the test using the hypophysectomized mouse as experimental model (Smith et al., 1982). This animal responds to Newcastle disease virus (NDV) infection with increased corticosterone production. Inasmuch as spleen cells of the virus-treated, hypophysectomized animal immunofluoresce with antibody to ACTH, in contrast to cells from control mice, the steroid response is presumably mediated by lymphocyte-derived ACTH (given the total absence of pituitary input).

These preliminary findings notwithstanding, the presumption that sensitized leukocytes can produce soluble proteins capable of mimicking the effects of a tropic, feedback-controlled pituitary hormone (i.e., ACTH) must remain a presumption, at least for the present. Contrary to the results reported by Blalock and his group, a 1983 study by Vahouny and colleagues showed neither evidence of increased corticosterone output by adrenal fasciculata cells, nor significant increase in cyclic AMP (cAMP) production in an ACTH-responsive adrenal membrane preparation, following their incubation in either thymic peptide, or lymphokine, medium.

Finally, it remains to be seen how a recently discovered lymphokine of impressive potency, "provisionally designated" glucocorticoid increasing factor (GIF), might be fitted into this developing mosaic (Besedovsky et al., 1985b). More powerful than ACTH, GIF increases ACTH and corticosterone output four-fold when systemically administered in the rat. The lymphokine effect is believed to be mediated through the pituitary, rather than the adrenal gland, in view of its complete elimination following dexamethasone treatment, a drug that blocks pituitary response.

THYMOSINS, CYTOKINES, AND THE CENTRAL NERVOUS SYSTEM

Interesting in themselves, these preceding observations are the more interesting when we take into account similarities between the thymosins, the lymphokines, and those peptides that are shown to be psychoactive. We will recall the comment by David L. Healy and associates (1983) that a "vasopressin-like amino acid sequence" might be responsible for the neuroendocrine activity of the thymus gland. The antidiuretic hormone (ADH), arginine vasopressin, is one such psychoactive peptide.

In effect, therefore, this single comment opens a window on a domain of biobehavioral research that has thus far remained conceptually disconnected from psychoneuroimmunology. In fact, when it can be claimed that thymosin peptides are neuromodulators (Hall et al., 1985a)—a claim in keeping with current reassessments in neuroscience—it would seem a violation of logic to ignore a research literature that describes, in meticulous detail, the physiologic and *psychologic* properties of that other peptide family, the opiomelanocortins.

Ablation and lesioning of selected brain areas, and the intracerebral injection and crystalline implantation of these latter peptides, and their secondary fragments, have been found to induce wide-ranging phar-macologic, behavioral, and cognitive effects. A partial listing of these ef-fects would include sedation, analgesia, amnesia, dysphoria, catatonia, retention and extinction behavior, memory consolidation and retrieval, ap-petitive acquisition, as well as active and passive avoidance learning (Bohus, 1984; de Weid & Jolles, 1982; Kastin et al., 1981; van Wimersma Greidanus et al., 1983).

As a leading investigator has observed: "how this multiplexity of infor-mation is 'extracted' from the precursor molecule under physiological cir-cumstances is not yet clear" (Bohus, 1984, p. 443). A first insight into the process comes of the discovery that, at least with respect to ACTH and beta-endorphin, specific (but again dissociated) endocrine and neuro-endocrine effects are mediated through five opiate receptor subtypes (mu, delta, kappa, sigma, epsilon) and their respective ligand specificities (Bohus, 1984; Copolov, 1985; Gispen et al., 1975; Zukin & Zukin, 1984).

In the hormone, arginine vasopressin, we have an excellent example of peptide "multiplexity." As its name implies, the hormone helps to maintain extracellular fluid and electrolyte balance by stimulating water reabsorp-tion from the renal tubules in near-perfect counterbalance to the diuretic, vasodilatory action of the cardiac (atrial) peptide hormone, atriopeptin (Manning et al., 1985). Vasopressin also acts as both releasing hormone and lymphokine. As releasing hormone, it stimulates the secretion of ad-renocorticotropin (ACTH) in synergism with corticoliberin (Rivier & Vale, 1983). As lymphokine, vasopressin replaces interleukin 2 (IL-2) in the production of gamma-interferon by T lymphocytes, *in vitro* (Johnson et al., 1982; Johnson & Torres, 1985). Lastly, in the form of a fragment es-sentially devoid of classic endocrine properties (de Wied & Bohus, 1979), vasopressin acts as psychoactive neuromodulator, facilitating vigilance, memory retrieval and storage, as well as affecting the emotions and drives that motivate avoidance behavior (van Wimersma Greidanus et al., 1983).

The story of the peptides, as it has unfolded from the perspective of immunology, underscores the fact that immune reactivity is intrinsic to the psychoneuroendocrine reaction patterns that characterize the stress response (Axelrod & Reisine, 1984)—a response, or set of responses, documented in countless multidisciplinary studies, utilizing countless ex-perimental "stress" paradigms. Now newly appreciated are the receptor-mediated processes carried out by peptides (Schmitt, 1984) that join together, in a synchronous network, the limbic forebrain—that central "node" critical to the mobilization of the emotions—and the peripheral or-gans, including the organs of immunity (Pert et al., 1985).

Peptide molecules share chemical, structural, and functional characteris-tics *across* systems. Consequently, it is not unlikely that thymosins, as members of this constellation of bioactive proteins, perform some of those functions attributed to related members of the group, and that they may do so within these same control centers of the brain. Like the opiomelanocortins, thymosin-, lymphocyte-, and monocyte-derived peptides exhibit functional specialization, said specialization differing as a function of tissue source: i.e., central (neuroendocrine), or peripheral (endocrine). It may yet be discovered that precision microinjection of immune system peptides, and their proteolytically-cleaved fragments, into selected target areas of the CNS can induce behavioral and mood effects of comparable specificity.

Information Processing in Local Circuits

Without unduly violating a concept that originated in a specialized area of neurophysiology, it is possible to ascribe the salient properties of what has been called "local circuitry" to non-neuronal cells, even to cells and molecules of the immune system. This "modulatory," "enabling" mode of cell:cell communication involves a form of signal exchange other than the spike-wave synaptic conduction of neuronal impulse. The interconnection of local circuit neurons is described as being dependent upon "small computational units or modules," desmosomes, serial and reciprocal synapses, uni- and bidirectional gap junctions, etc. (Rakic, 1975; Schmitt, Dev, & Smith, 1976; Sloper, 1972; Sotelo, 1977).

Peptide-secreting cells impact on other central neurons in ways that resemble local circuitry (Barker et al., 1978). McCulloch (1984) has observed the "unusual anatomical arrangements between the brain and its vasculature," which allow peptidergic neurons to come into "intimate, direct contact" with the cerebral microcirculation (p. 135). It is also possible that peptide cells in the vertebrate brain, like those in invertebrates (e.g., *Aplysia*), utilize the extracellular matrix as medium for nonsynaptic signal transmission (Mayeri & Rothman, 1981).

The behavior of certain brain cells, other than neurons, suggests junctional mediation of the "enabling" mode. Ependymocytes (neuroglia) are specialized pleomorphic, phagocytic cells that line the inner surface of the third ventricle immediately adjacent to the paraventricular nucleus of the hypothalamus (Brawer & Walsh, 1982). Junctions between ependyma dispersed throughout the median eminence and the infundibular zone act as differentially permeable barriers to the movement of hormonal substances (Monroe & Holmes, 1982) and permit the intercellular flux of negatively-charged polypeptides (Bennet, Spray, & Harris, 1981). It is believed that ependymocytes selectively facilitate the transport of biologically active materials between hypothalamus, cerebrospinal fluid, and the circulatory network of the anterior pituitary (Bleier, 1972; Pilgrim, 1978; Porter et al., 1975) and guide, as well, their retrograde movement along this same corridor (Dorsa et al., 1981).

Otherwise, the hypothalamus and the pituitary gland contain high concentrations of perivascular satellite cells, or microglia, as defined immunohistochemically by the macrophage-specific glycoprotein antigen, F4/80 (Hume et al., 1984). Contrary to common belief, glial cells are excitable. Their plasma membranes contain voltage-sensitive ion channels, implying the presence of uptake and/or transport mechanisms for transmitters, and other small molecules (Gray & Ritchie, 1985). As N. Joan Abbott (1985) has put it, microglia may have been presumed "silent" only "because we aren't clever enough to hear them talking" (p. 142). Now, with the microelectrode probe and the patch electrode—this last recording currents as minuscule as a few picoamperes—we may be recording "the first whispers."

The microcircuitry of glia, i.e., the circuits they help to support, and the inputs to which they might be subject from the surrounding medium and the activity of neighboring cells, has hardly begun to be defined. Evidence is sketchy, at best suggestive. It is known that glia, like peripheral macrophages, secrete high titers of an interleukin 1-like soluble factor (Fontana et al., 1982), which stimulates ACTH release, in vitro (Woloski et al., 1985). In turn, we may deduce that the central migration of microglia might be stimulated by opioid peptides, in view of evidence that chemotaxis in peripheral mononuclear cells is so influenced, in vitro (Ruff et al., 1985; van Epps & Saland, 1984).

Finally, it is conceivable that lymphokine molecules of peripheral origin, having gained access to the brain through the infundibular pathway, might influence brain cells by local mediation. One possible mechanism of influence may rest in the fact that the lymphokine, interferon, is capable of inducing the transfer of viral resistance to receptor-less cells, in vitro, presumably by gap junction and the transfer of second messenger molecules (e.g., cyclic AMP) (Blalock & Baron, 1977).

CONCLUSIONS

It has been argued that the modern day concept of physiologic systems is an arbitrary one—an inevitable reflection of our self-perspective as evolved vertebrates, but arbitrary, nonetheless. As a consequence of this bias, our conceptual approach to the study of biologic systems has been termed *neurocentric* (Roth et al., 1985). To account, for example, for the appearance of the neuropeptides (an "event" of the 1940s, heralded by the discovery of the hypothalamic secretory cell by Ernst and Bertha Scharrer [1940]), theories were advanced that would show these cells to have been evolutionary latecomers, derivatives of neural tissue (Pearse, 1969, 1981), which they are not.

In direct contradiction to the neurocentric view, the proposed *paleocentric* view would acknowledge the ancient history and ubiquity of peptides. It would call attention to their long evolution in the biosphere, mark their presence (and that of their receptors) in a wide variety of cell types, and appreciate their structural and functional relatedness, whether isolated from human brain, the tissues of unicellular organisms, or the cells of the higher plants (Doolittle, 1984; LeRoith, Shiloach, & Roth, 1982; Roth et al., 1982, 1983, 1985).

In this chapter, we have followed the efforts of scientists who seek to understand relationships and interactions between three principal physiological systems of the body. We have noted some of the private (unique), as well as the surprisingly numerous public (common), mediums of communication used by these systems. We will also have noted that, when subjected to review, published reports on aspects of systems interaction hardly present a synthesis. Perhaps a broader approach to the study of peptides—an ecology of peptides, so to speak—would produce a perspective on biological systems that would allow for a more harmonious arrangement of the facts.

If, on the basis of an evolutionary perspective, systems, as such, were to be understood as "novel," as having been imposed, in recent time, upon molecular networks of communication extant from earliest time, our present semantic and conceptual difficulties might be eased. We would realize that systems are intricately specialized biological entities, made separate under the relentless strictures of evolution. We would also understand that, to remain viable, they must continue to utilize still other biological entities of infinitely more ancient and universal origin.

REFERENCES

Abbott, N. J. Are glial cells excitable after all? *Trends in Neurosciences*, 1985, 8 (4), 141-142.

Agnati, L. F., Fuxe, K., Locatelli, V., Benfenati, F., Zini, I., Panerai, A. E., El Etreby, M. F., & Hökfelt, T. Neuroanatomical methods for the quantitative evaluation of coexistence of transmitters in nerve cells. Analysis of the ACTH- and β-endorphin immunoreactive nerve cell bodies of the mediobasal hypothalamus of the rat. *Journal of Neuroscience Methods,* 1982, 5 (3), 203-214.

Anschel, S., Alexander, M., & Perachio, A. A. Multiple connections of medial hypothalamic neurons in the rat. *Experimental Brain Research,* 1982, 46 (3), 383-392.

Axelrod, J., & Reisine, T. D. Stress hormones: Their interaction and regulation. *Science,* 1984, 224 (4648), 452-459.

Barchas, J. D., Akil, H., Elliott, G. R., Holman, R. B., & Watson, S. J. Behavioral neurochemistry: Neuroregulators and behavioral states. *Science,* 1978, 200 (4344), 964-973.

Barker, J. L., Neale, J. H., Smith T. G., & MacDonald, R. L. Opiate peptide modulation of amino acid responses suggests novel form of neuronal communication. *Science,* 1978, 199 (4336), 1451-1453.

Beinfeld, M. C., Lewis, M. E., Eiden, L. E., Nilaver, G., & Pert, C. B. The distribution of cholecystokinin and vasoactive intestinal peptide in rhesus monkey brain as determined by radioimmunoassay. *Neuropeptides,* 1983, 3 (5), 337-344.

Bennett, M. V. L., Spray, D. C., & Harris, A. L. Gap junctions and development. *Trends in Neurosciences,* 1981, 4, 159-163.

Bergland, R. M., Blume, H., Hamilton, A., Monica, P., & Patterson, R. Adrenocorticotropic hormone may be transported directly from the pituitary to the brain. *Science,* 1980, 210 (4469), 541-543.

Bergland, R. M., & Page, R. B. Pituitary-brain vascular relations: A new paradigm. *Science,* 1979, 204 (4388), 18-24.

Besedovsky, H., & Sorkin, E. Network of immune-neuroendocrine interactions. *Clinical and Experimental Immunology,* 1977, 27 (1), 1-12.

Besedovsky, H., del Rey, A., & Sorkin, E. Lymphokine containing supernatants from Con A-stimulated cells increase corticosterone blood levels. *Journal of Immunology,* 1981, 126 (1), 385-387.

Besedovsky, H., del Rey, A, & Sorkin, E. Immunological-neuroendocrine feedback circuits. In R. Guillemin, M. Cohn, & T. Melnechuck (Eds.), *Neural Modulation of Immunity.* New York: Raven Press, 1985a, 165-172.

Besedovsky, H., del Rey, A., Sorkin, E., & Dinarello, C. A. Immunoregulatory feedback between interleukin-1 and glucocorticoid hormones. *Science,* 1986, 233 (4764), 652-654.

Besedovsky, H., del Rey, A., Sorkin, E., Lotz, W., & Schwulera, U. Lymphoid cells produce an immunoregulatory glucocorticoid increasing factor (GIF) acting through the pituitary gland. *Clinical and Experimental Immunology,* 1985b, 59 (3), 622-628.

Besedovsky, H. O., del Rey, A., Sorkin, E., DaPrada, M., Burri, R., & Honegger, C. The immune response evokes changes in brain noradrenergic neurons. *Science,* 1983, 221 (4610), 564-566.

Besedovsky, H. O., Sorkin, E., Felix, D., & Haas, H. Hypothalamic changes during the immune response. *European Journal of Immunology,* 1977, 7 (5), 325-328.

Bhathena, S. J., Louie, J., Schechter, G. P., Redman, R. S., Wahl, L., & Recant, L. Identification of human mononuclear leukocytes bearing receptors for somatostatin and glucagon. *Diabetes,* 1981, 30 (2), 127-131.

Blalock, J. E. The immune system as a sensory organ. *Journal of Immunology,* 1984a, 132 (3), 1067-1070.

Blalock, J. E. Relationships between neuroendocrine hormones and lymphokines. In E. Pick (Ed.), *Lymphokines: A Forum for Immunoregulatory Cell Products,* Vol. 9. New York: Academic Press, 1984b, 1-13.

Blalock, J. E., & Baron, S. Interferon-induced transfer of viral resistance between animal cells. *Nature (London),* 1977, 269 (5627), 422-425.

Blalock, J. E., Harbour-McMenamin, D., & Smith, E. M. Peptide hormones shared by the neuroendocrine and immunologic systems. *Journal of Immunology,* 1985, 135 (2 Suppl.), 858s-861s.

Blalock, J. E., & Harp, C. Interferon and adrenocorticotropic hormone induction of steroidogenesis, melanogenesis, and antiviral activity. *Archives of Virology,* 1981, 67 (1), 45-49.

Blalock, J. E., & Smith, E. M. A complete regulatory loop between the immune and neuroendocrine systems. *Federation Proceedings,* 1985, 44 (1, pt. 1), 108-111.

Bleier, R. Structural relationship of ependymal cells and their processes within the hypothalamus: Implications for functional localization. In K. M. Knigge, D. E. Scott, & A. Weindl (Eds.), *International Symposium on Brain-Endocrine Interaction (1971: Munich). Brain-Endocrine Interaction. Median Eminence: Structure and Function.* Basel: S. Karger, 1972, 306-318.

Bloom, F. E., Battenberg, E. L., Rivier, J., & Vale, W. Corticotropin releasing factor (CRF): Immunoreactive neurones and fibers in rat hypothalamus. *Regulatory Peptides,* 1982, 4 (1), 43-48.

Bockman, D. E., & Kirby, M. L. Neural crest interactions in the development of the immune system. *Journal of Immunology,* 1985, 135 (2 Suppl.), 766s-768s.

Bohus, B. Opiomelanocortins and behavioral adaptation. *Pharmacology and Therapeutics,* 1984, 26 (3), 417-451.

Brawer, J. R., & Walsh, R. J. Response of tanycytes to aging in the median eminence of the rat. *American Journal of Anatomy,* 1982, 163 (3), 247-256.

Brownstein, M. J., Russell, J. T., & Gainer, H. Synthesis, transport, and release of posterior pituitary hormones. *Science,* 1980, 207 (4429), 373-378.

Bulloch, K., & Moore, R. Y. Innervation of the thymus gland by brainstem and spinal cord in mouse and rat. *American Journal of Anatomy,* 1981, 162 (2), 157-166.

Chany, C., Rousset, S., Bourgeade, M. F., Mathieu, D., & Grégoire, A. Role of receptors and the cytoskeleton in reverse transformation and steroidogenesis induced by interferon. *Annals of the New York Academy of Sciences,* 1980, 350, 254-265.

Chrétien, M., Benjannet, S., Gossard, F., Gianoulakis, C., Crine, P., Lis, M., & Seidah, N. G. From beta-lipotropin to beta-endorphin and 'pro-opio-melanocortin.' *Canadian Journal of Biochemistry,* 1979, 57 (9), 1111-1121.

Cohen, S. N., Chang, A. C., Nakanishi, S., Inoue, A., Kita, T., Nakamura, M., & Numa, S. Studies of cloned DNA encoding the structure for the bovine corticotropin-beta-lipotropin precursor protein. *Annals of the New York Academy of Sciences,* 1980, 343, 415-424.

Cooper, E. L. *General Immunology.* 1st edition. New York: Pergamon Press, 1982.

Copolov, D. L. Opioid biology: The next set of questions. *Australian and New Zealand Journal of Medicine (Sydney),* 1985, 15 (1), 98-106.

Cross, R. J., Markesbery, W. R., Brooks, W. H., & Roszman, T. L. Hypothalamic-immune interaction. I. The acute effect of anterior hypothalamic lesions on the immune response. *Brain Research,* 1980, 196 (1), 79-87.

Crotti, A. *Thyroid and Thymus.* Philadelphia: Lea & Febiger, Publishers, 1918.

Cummings, S., Elde, R., Ells, J., & Lindall, A. Corticotropin-releasing factor immunoreactivity is widely distributed within the central nervous system of the rat: An immunohistochemical study. *Journal of Neuroscience,* 1983, 3 (7), 1355-1368.

Danek, A., O'Dorisio, M. S., O'Dorisio, T. M., & George, J. M. Specific binding sites for vasoactive intestinal polypeptide on nonadherent peripheral blood lymphocytes. *Journal of Immunology,* 1983, 131 (3), 1173-1177.

Defendini, R., & Zimmerman, E. A. The magnocellular neurosecretory system of the mammalian hypothalamus. In S. Reichlin, R. J. Baldessarini, & J. B. Martin (Eds.), *The Hypothalamus. Research Publications: Association for Research in Nervous and Mental Diseases,* Vol. 56. New York: Raven Press, 1978, 56:137-154.

de Kloet, R., Veldhuis, D., & Bohus, B. Significance of neuropeptides in the control of corticosterone-receptor activity in rat brain. In G. C. Pepeu, M. J. Kuhar, & S. J. Enna (Eds.), *International Colloquium on Receptors, Neurotransmitters and peptide hormones (1st: 1979: Capri). Receptors for Neurotransmitters and Peptide Hormones. Advances in Biochemical Psychopharmacology,* Vol. 21. New York: Raven Press, 1980, 373-382.

de Wied, D., & Bohus, B. Modulation of memory processes by neuropeptides of hypothalamic-neurohypophyseal origin. In M. A. Brazier (Ed.), *Brain Mechanisms in Memory and Learning: From the Single Neuron to Man.*

New York: Raven Press, 1979, 139-149.

de Wied, D., & Jolles, J. Neuropeptides derived from pro-opiocortin: Behavioral, physiological and neurochemical effects. *Physiological Reviews,* 1982, 62 (3), 976-1059.

Docherty, K., & Steiner, D. F. Post-translational proteolysis in polypeptide hormone biosynthesis. *Annual Review of Physiology,* 1982, 44, 625-638.

Doolittle, R. F. Protein evolution: Modern proteins with ancient roots. *Federation Proceedings,* 1984, 43 (6), 1669. (Symposium abstr. No. 1477)

Dorsa, D. M., de Kloet, E. R., van Dijk, A. M. J., & Mezey, E. Retrograde transport of neuropeptides as a pituitary-brain communication system. In D. S. Farner & K. Lederis (Eds.), *International Symposium on Neurosecretion (8th: 1980: Friday Harbor, Washington). Neurosecretion: Molecules, Cells, Systems.* New York: Plenum Press, 1981, 197-209.

Dunn, A. J., & Gispen, W. H. How ACTH acts on the brain. *Biobehavioral Reviews,* 1977, 1 (1), 15-23.

Eipper, B. A., & Mains, R. E. Existence of a common precursor to ACTH and endorphin in the anterior and intermediate lobe of the rat pituitary. *Journal of Supramolecular Structure,* 1978, 8 (3), 247-262.

Eipper, B. A., & Mains, R. E. Structure and biosynthesis of pro-adrenocorticotropin/endorphin and related peptides. *Endocrinology Review,* 1980, 1 (1), 1-27.

Felten, D. L., Felten, S. Y., Carlson, S. L., Olschowka, J. A., & Livnat, S. Noradrenergic and peptidergic innervation of lymphoid tissue. *Journal of Immunology,* 1985, 135 (2 Suppl.), 755s-765s.

Fontana, A., Kristensen, F., Dubs, R., Gemsa, D., & Weber, E. Production of prostaglandin E and an interleukin-1 like factor by cultured astrocytes and C6 glioma cells. *Journal of Immunology,* 1982, 129 (6), 2413-2419.

Fujiwara, M., Muryobayashi, T., & Shimamoto, K. Histochemical demonstration of monoamines in the thymus of rats. *Japanese Journal of Pharmacology,* 1966, 16 (4), 493-494.

Gagner, J. P., & Drouin, J. Opposite regulation of pro-opiomelanocortin gene transcription by glucocorticoids and CRH. *Molecular and Cellular Endocrinology,* 1985, 40 (1), 25-32.

Gaudreau, P., St. Pierre, S., Pert, C. B., & Quirion, R. Cholecystokinin receptors in mammalian brain. A comparative characterization and visualization. *Annals of the New York Academy of Sciences,* 1985, 448, 198-219.

Gavin, J. R., III, Gordon, P., Roth, J., Archer, J. A., & Buell, D. N. Characteristics of the human lymphocyte insulin receptor. *Journal of Biological Chemistry,* 1973, 248 (6), 2202-2207.

Geenen, V., Legros, J. J., Franchimont, P., Baudrihaye, M., Defresne, M. P., & Boniver, J. The neuroendocrine thymus: Coexistence of oxytocin and neurophysin in the human thymus. *Science,* 1986, 232 (4749), 508-511.

Giron, L. T., Crutcher, K. A., & Davis, J. N. Lymph nodes—A possible site for sympathetic neuronal regulation of immune responses. *Annals of Neurology,* 1980, 8 (5), 520-525.

Gispen, W. H., Wiegant, V. M., Greven, H. M., & de Wied, D. The induction of excessive grooming in the rat by intraventricular application of peptides derived from ACTH: Structure-activity studies. *Life Science,* 1975, 17 (4), 645-652.

Goldstein, A., & Ghazarossian, V. E. Immunoreactive dynorphin in pituitary and brain. *Proceedings of the National Academy of Sciences, U.S.A.,* 1980, 77 (10), 6207-6210.

Goldstein, A. L., Low, T. L., McAdoo, M., McClure, J., Thurman, G. B., Rossio, J., Lai, C. Y., Chang, D., Wang, S. S., Harvey, C., Ramel, A. H., & Meienhofer, J. Thymosin alpha 1: Isolation and sequence analysis of an immunologically active thymic polypeptide. *Proceedings of the National Academy of Sciences, U.S.A.,* 1977, 74 (2), 725-729.

Gray, P. T. A., & Ritchie, J. M. Ion channels in Schwann and glial cells. *Trends in Neurosciences*, 1985, 8 (9), 411-415.

Guillemin, R., Vargo, T., Rossier, J., Minick, S., Ling, N., Rivier, C., Vale, W., & Bloom, F. β-Endorphin and adrenocorticotropin are secreted concomitantly by the pituitary gland. *Science,* 1977, 197 (4311), 1367-1369.

Hall, N. R., McGillis, J. P., Spangelo, B. L., Palaszynski, E., Moody, T. W., & Goldstein, A. L. Evidence for a neuroendocrine-thymus axis mediated by thymosin polypeptides. In B. Serrou, C. Rosenfeld, J. C. Daniels, & J. P. Saunders (Eds.), *Current Concepts in Human Immunology and Cancer Immunomodulation.* New York: Elsevier/North Holland, 1982, 653-660.

Hall, N. R., McGillis, J. P., Spangelo, B. L., & Goldstein, A. L. Evidence that thymosins and other biologic response modifiers can function as neuroactive immunotransmitters. *Journal of Immunology,* 1985a, 135 (2 Suppl.), 806s-811s.

Hall, N. R., McGillis, J. P., Spangelo, B. L., Healy, D. L., Chrousos, G. P., Schulte, H. M., & Goldstein, A. L. Thymic hormone effect on the brain and neuroendocrine circuits. In R. Guillemin, M. Cohn, & T. Melnechuk (Eds.), *Neural Modulation of Immunity.* New York: Raven Press, 1985b, 179-190.

Hammar, J. A. Konstitutionsanatomische Studien über die Neurotisierung des Menschenembryos: Über die Innervationsverhaltnisse der Inkretorgane und der Thymus bis in den 4. Fötalmonat. *Zeitschrift für Microskopisch-anatomische Forschung,* 1935, 38, 253-293.

Hazum, E., Chang, K. J., & Cuatrecasas, P. Specific nonopiate receptors for beta-endorphin. *Science,* 1979, 205 (4410), 1033-1035.

Healy, D. L., Hodgen, G. D., Schulte, H. M., Chrousos, G. P., Loriaux, D. L., Hall, N. R., & Goldstein, A. L. The thymus-adrenal connection: Thymosin has corticotropin-releasing activity in primates. *Science,* 1983, 222 (4630), 1353-1355.

Horecker, B. L., & Morgan, J. Ubiquitous distribution of thymosin 4 and related peptides in vertebrate cells and tissues. In E. Pike (Ed.), *Lymphokines: A Forum for Immunoregulatory Products,* Vol. 9. New York: Academic Press, 1984, 15-35.

Hume, D. A., Halpin, D., Charlton, H., & Gordon, S. The mononuclear phagocytic system of the mouse defined by immunohistochemical localization of antigen F4/80: Macrophages of endocrine organs. *Proceedings of the National Academy of Sciences, U.S.A.,* 1984, 81 (13), 4174-4177.

Johnson, H. M., Farrer, W. L., & Torres, B. A. Vasopressin replacement of interleukin 2 requirement in gamma interferon production: Lymphokine activity of a neuroendocrine hormone. *Journal of Immunology,* 1982,129 (3), 983-986.

Johnson, H. M., & Torres, B. A. Regulation of lymphokine production by arginine vasopressin and oxytocin: Modulation of lymphocyte function by neurohypophysial hormones. *Journal of Immunology,* 1985, 135 (2 Suppl.), 773s-775s.

Jones, M. T., Gillham, B., Greenstein, B. D., Beckford, U., & Holmes, M. C. Feedback actions of adrenal steroid hormones. In D. Ganten & D. Pfaff (Eds.), *Adrenal Actions on Brain.* New York: Springer-Verlag, 1982, 45-68.

Jones, M. T., Hillhouse, E. W., & Burden, J. Effect on various putative neurotransmitters on the secretion of corticotropin-releasing hormone from the rat hypothalamus in vitro: A model of the neurotransmitters involved. *Journal of Endocrinology,* 1976, 69 (1), 1-10.

Joseph, S. A., & Knigge, K. M. The endocrine hypothalamus: Recent anatomical studies. *Research Publications: Association for Research in Nervous and Mental Diseases,* 1978, 56, 15-47.

Kastin, A. J., Olson, R. D., Sandman, C. A., & Coy, D. H. Multiple independent action of neuropeptides on behavior. In J. L. Martinez, Jr., R. A. Jensen, R. B. Messing, H. Rigter, & J. L. McCaugh (Eds.), *Endogenous Peptides and Learning and Memory Processes.* New York: Academic Press, 1981, 563-577.

Kobayashi, H., Matsui, T., & Ishii, S. Functional electron microscopy of the hypothalamic median eminence. *International Review of Cytology,* 1970, 29, 281-381.

Kordon, C., Enjalbert, A., Epelbaum, J., & Rotsztejn, W. Neurotransmitter interactions with adenohypophyseal regulation. In A. M. Gotto, Jr., E. J. Peck, Jr., & A. E. Boyd, III (Eds.), *Argenteuil Symposium (4th: 1978: Waterloo, Belgium). Brain Peptides: A New Endocrinology.* New York: Elsevier/North-Holland Biomedical Press, 1979, 277-293.

LeRoith, D., Shiloach, J., & Roth, J. Is there an earlier phylogenetic precursor that is common to both the nervous and endocrine systems? *Peptides (Fayetteville), 1982, 3 (3), 211-215.*

Liotta, A. S., Gildersleeve, D., Brownstein, M. J., & Krieger, D. T. Biosynthesis in vitro of immunoreactive 31,000 dalton corticotropin/β-endorphin-like material by bovine hypothalamus. *Proceedings of the National Academy of Sciences, U.S.A.*, 1979, 76 (3), 1448-1452.

Lloyd, R. Mechanisms of psychoneuroimmunological response. In B. H. Fox, & B. H. Newberry (Eds.), *Impact of Psychoendocrine Systems in Cancer and Immunity.* Toronto: C. J. Hogrefe, Inc., 1984, 1-57.

Löfgren, F. New aspects of the hypothalamic control of the adenohypophysis. *Acta Morphological Neerlando-Scandinavica,* 1959a, 2, 220-229.

Löfgren, F. The infundibular recess: A component of the hypothalamo-adreno-hypophyseal system. *Acta Morphologica Neerlando-Scandinavica,* 1959b, 3, 55-78.

Low, T. L., Thurman, G. B., McAdoo, M., McClure, J. E., Rossio, J. L., Naylor, P. H., & Goldstein, A. L. The chemistry and biology of thymosin. I. Isolation, characterization, and biological activities of thymosin alpha1 and polypeptide 1 from calf thymus. *Journal of Biological Chemistry,* 1979, 254 (3), 981-986.

Mains, R. E., Eipper, B. A., & Ling, N. Common precursor to corticotropins and endorphins. *Proceedings of the National Academy of Sciences, U.S.A.,* 1977, 74 (7), 3014-3018.

Manning, P. T., Schwartz, D., Katsube, N. C., Holmberg, S. W., & Needleman, P. Vasopressin-stimulated release of atriopeptin: Endocrine antagonists in fluid homeostasis. *Science,* 1985, 229 (4711), 395-397.

Maśliński, W., Grabcżewska, E., & Ryzewski, J. Acetylcholine receptors of rat lymphocytes. *Biochimica et Biophysica Acta,* 1980, 633 (2), 269-273.

Mathison, J. C., Schreiber, R. D., La Forest, A. C., & Ulevitch, R. J. Suppression of ACTH-induced steroidogenesis by supernatants from LPS-treated peritoneal exudate macrophages. *Journal of Immunology,* 1983, 130, (6), 2757-2762.

Mayeri, E., & Rothman, B. S. Nonsynaptic peptidergic neurotransmission in the abdominal ganglion of *Aplysia*. In D. S. Farner & K. Lederis (Eds.), *Eighth International Symposium on Neurosecretion (8th: 1980: Friday Harbor, Washington). Neurosecretion: Molecules, cells, systems.* New York: Plenum Press, 1981, 305-316.

Mayr, E. Evolution. *Scientific American,* 1978, 239,(3), 46-55.

McCulloch, J. Perivascular nerve fibers and the cerebral circulation. *Trends in Neurosciences,* 1984, 7 (5), 135-138.

McGillis, J. P., Hall, N. R., Vahouny, G. V., & Goldstein, A. L. Thymosin fraction 5 causes increased serum corticosterone in rodents in vivo. *The Journal of Immunology,* 1985, 134 (6), 3952-3955.

Monroe, B. G., & Holmes, E. M. The freeze-fractured median eminence. I. Development of intercellular junctions in the ependyma of the 3rd ventricle of the rat. *Cell Tissue Research,* 1982, 222 (2), 389-408.

Palaszynski, E. W., Moody, T. W., O'Donohue, T. L., & Goldstein, A. L. Thymosin alpha1-like peptides: Localization and biochemical characterization in the rat brain and pituitary gland. *Peptides* (Fayetteville), 1983, 4 (4), 463-467.

Payan, D. G., Brewster, D. R., & Goetzl, E. J. Stereospecific receptors for substance P on cultured human IM-9 lymphoblasts. *Journal of Immunology,* 1984, 133 (6), 3260-3265.

Pearse, A. G. E. The cytochemistry and ultrastructure of polypeptide hormone-producing cells of the APUD series, and the embryologic, physiological and pathologic implications of the concept. *Journal of Histochemistry and Cytochemistry,* 1969, 17 (5), 303-313.

Pearse, A. G. E. Molecular markers and the APUD concept. In D. S. Farner, & K. Lederis (Eds.), *International Symposium on Neurosecretion (8th: 1980: Friday Harbor, Washington). Neurosecretion: Molecules, Cells, Systems.* New York: Plenum Press, 1981, 15-28.

Pelletier, G. Ultrastructural localization of a fragment (16K) of the common precursor for adrenocorticotropin (ACTH) and β-lipotropin (β-LPH) in the rat hypothalamus. *Neuroscience Letter,* 1980, 16 (1), 85-90.

Pert, C. B., Ruff, M. R., Weber, R. J., & Herkenham, M. Neuropeptides and their receptors: A psychosomatic network. *Journal of Immunology,* 1985, 135 (2 Suppl.), 820s-826s.

Pictet, R. L., Rall, L. B., Phelps, P., & Rutter, W. J. The neural crest and the origin of the insulin-producing and other gastrointestinal hormone-producing cells. *Science,* 1976, 191 (4223), 191-192.

Pilgrim, C. Transport function of hypothalamic tanycyte ependyma: How good is the evidence? *Neuroscience,* 1978, 3 (3), 277-283.

Pochet, R., Delespesse, G., Gausset, P. W., & Collet, H. Distribution of beta-adrenergic receptors on human lymphocyte subpopulations. *Clinical & Experimental Immunology,* 1979, 38 (3), 578-584.

Porter, J. C., Ben-Jonathan, N., Oliver, C., & Eskay, R. L. Secretion of releasing hormones and their transport from CSF to hypophysial portal blood. In K. M. Knigge, D. E. Scott, H. Kobayashi, & S. Ishii (Eds.), *International Symposium on Brain-Endocrine Interaction (2nd: 1974: Schizuoka). Brain-endocrine interaction. II. The ventricular system in neuroendocrine mechanisms.* Basel: S. Karger, 1975, 295-305.

Rakic, P. Local circuit neurons. *Neuroscience Research Program Bulletin,* 1975, 13 (3), 295-416.

Rayford, P. L., Miller, T. A., & Thompson, J. C. Secretin, cholecystokinin and newer gastrointestinal hormones (first of two parts). *New England Journal of Medicine,* 1976a, 294 (20), 1093-1101.

Rayford, P. L., Miller, T. A., & Thompson, J. C. Secretin, cholecystokinin and newer gastrointestinal hormones (second of two parts). *New England Journal of Medicine,* 1976b, 294 (21), 1157-1163.

Rebar, R. W., Miyake, A., Low, T. L. K., & Goldstein, A. L. Thymosin stimulates secretion of luteinizing hormone-releasing factor. *Science,* 1981, 214 (4521), 669-671.

Reilly, F. D., McCuskey, P. A., Miller, M. L., McCuskey, R. S., & Meineke, H. A. Innervation of the periarteriolar lymphatic sheath of the spleen. *Tissue Cell,* 1979, 11 (1), 121-126.

Renaud, L. P., Pittman, Q. J., & Blume, H. W. Neurophysiology of hypothalamic peptidergic neurons. In K. Fuxe, T. Hökfelt, & R. Luft (Eds.), *Central Regulation of the Endocrine System.* New York: Plenum Press, 1979, 119-136.

Rivier, C., & Vale, W. Interaction of corticotropin-releasing factor and arginine vasopressin on adrenocorticotropin secretion in vivo. *Endocrinology,* 1984, 113 (3), 934-942.

Roberts, J. L., & Herbert, E. Characterization of common precursor to corticotropin and β-lipotropin: Cell-free synthesis of the precursor and identification of corticotropin peptides in the molecule. *Proceedings of the National Academy of Sciences, U.S.A.,* 1977a, 74 (11), 4826-4830.

Roberts, J. L., & Herbert, E. Characterization of a common precursor to corticotropin and β-lipotropin: Identification of β-lipotropin peptides and their arrangement relative to corticotropin in the precursor synthesized in a cell-free system. *Proceedings of the National Academy of Sciences, U.S.A.,* 1977b, 74 (12), 5300-5304.

Roszman, T. L., Cross, R. J., Brooks, W. H., & Markesbery, W. R. Hypothalamic-immune interaction. II. The effect of hypothalamic lesions on the ability of adherent spleen cells to limit lymphocyte blastogenesis. *Immunology,* 1982, 45 (4), 737-742.

Roszman, T. L., Jackson, J. C., Cross, R. J., Titus, M. J., Markesbery, W. R., & Brooks, W. H. Neuroanatomic and neurotransmitter influences on immune function. *Journal of Immunology,* 1985, 135 (2 Suppl.), 769s-772s.

Roth, J., LeRoith, D., Collier, E. S., Weaver, N. R., Watkinson, A., Cleland, C. F., & Glick, S. M. Evolutionary origins of neuropeptides, hormones, and receptors: Possible applications to immunology. *Journal of Immunology,* 1985, 135 (2 Suppl.), 816s-819s.

Roth, J., LeRoith, D., Shiloach, J., Rosenzweig, J. L., Lesniak, M. A., & Havrankova, J. The evolutionary origins of hormones, neurotransmitters, and other extracellular chemical messengers: Implications for mammalian biology. *New England Journal of Medicine,* 1982, 306 (9), 523-527.

Roth, J., LeRoith, D., Shiloach, J., & Tubinovitz, C. Intercellular communication: An attempt at a unifying hypothesis. *Clinical Research,* 1983, 31 (3), 354-363.

Rotsztejn, W. H. Neuromodulation in neuroendocrinology. *Trends in Neuroscience,* 1980, 3, 67-70.

Ruff, M. R., Wahl, S. M., Mergenhagen, S., & Pert, C. B. Opiate receptor-mediated chemotaxis of human monocytes. *Neuropeptides,* 1985, 5 (4-6), 363-366.

Said, S. I. Peptides common to the nervous system and the gastrointestinal tract. In L. Martini & W. F. Ganong (Eds.), *Frontiers in Neuroendocrinology,* Vol. 6. New York: Raven Press, 1980, 293-331.

Scharrer, E., & Scharrer, B. Secretory cells within the hypothalamus. *Research Publications. Proceedings (1939), Association for Research in Nervous and Mental Diseases,* Vol. 20. *The Hypothalamus and Central Levels of Autonomic Function.* New York: Raven Press, 1940, 170-194.

Schmitt, F. O. Molecular regulators of brain function: A new view. *Neuroscience,* 1984, 13 (4), 991-1001.

Schmitt, F. O., Dev, P., & Smith, B. H. Electrotonic processing of information by brain cells. *Science,* 1976, 193 (4248), 114-120.

Siggins, G. R. Modulators, mediators, and specifiers in brain function: Interactions of neuropeptides, cyclic nucleotides, and phosphoproteins in mechanisms underlying neuronal activity, behavior, and neuropsychiatric disorders. In Y. H. Ehrlich, J. Volavka, L. G. Davis, & E. G. Brungraber (Eds.), *Advances in Experimental Medicine and Biology,* Vol. 116. New York: Plenum Press, 1978, 41-64.

Sloper, J. J. Gap junctions between dendrites in the primate neocortex. *Brain Research,* 1972, 44 (2), 641-646.

Smith, E. M., & Blalock, J. E. Human lymphocyte production of corticotropin and endorphin-like substances: Association with leukocyte interferon. *Proceedings of the National Academy of Sciences, U.S.A.,* 1981, 78 (12), 7530-7534.

Smith, E. M., Harbour-McMenamin, D., & Blalock, J. E. Lymphocyte production of endorphins and endorphin-mediated immunoregulatory activity. *Journal of Immunology,* 1985, 135 (2 Suppl.), 779s-782s.

Smith, E. M., Johnson, H. M., & Blalock, J. E. Lymphocytes as a peripheral source of and target for endogenous opiates. In F. Fraioli, A. Isidori, & M. Mazzetti (Eds.), *International Symposium on Opioid Peptides in the Periphery (1984: Rome). Opioid Peptides in the Periphery.* New York: Elsevier Science Publishers, 1984, 129-136.

Smith, E. M., Meyer, W. J., & Blalock, J. E. Virus-induced corticosterone in hypophysectomized mice: A possible lymphoid adrenal axis. *Science,* 1982, 218 (4579), 1311-1312.

Smith, E. M., Phan, M., Kruger, T. E., Coppenhaver, D., & Blalock, J. E. Human lymphocyte production of immunoreactive thyrotropin. *Proceedings of the National Academy of Sciences, U.S.A.,* 1983, 80 (19), 6010-6013.

Sotelo, C. Electrical and chemical communication in the central nervous system. In B. R. Brinkley, & K. R. Porter (Eds.), *International Congress on Cell Biology (1st: 1976: Boston)*. *International Cell Biology*. New York: The Rockefeller University Press, 1977, 83-92.

Spector, N. H. (Editor-in-Chief), Bulloch, K., Fox, B. H., Janković, B. D., Kerza-Kwiatecki, A. P., Monjan, A. A., & Pierpaoli, W. (Assoc. Eds.), *International Workshop on Neuroimmunomodulation (1st: 1984: Bethesda, Maryland)*. Bethesda: International Working Group on Neuroimmunomodulation, 1986.

Spector, N. H., & Korneva, E. A. Neurophysiology, immunophysiology, and neuroimmunomodulation. In R. Ader (Ed.), *Psychoneuroimmunology*. New York: Academic Press, 1981, 449-473.

Stein, M., Schleifer, S. J., & Keller, S. E. Hypothalamic influence on immune responses. R. Ader (Ed.), *Psychoneuroimmunology*. New York: Academic Press, 1981, 429-447.

Stepién, H., Kunert-Radek, J., Karasek, E., & Pawlikowski, M. Dopamine increases cyclic AMP concentration in the rat spleen lymphocytes in vitro. *Biochemical and Biophysical Research Communications,* 1981, 101 (3), 1057-1063.

Vahouny, G. V., Kyeyune-Nyombi, E., McGillis, J. P., Tare, N. A., Huage, K. Y., Tombes, R., Goldstein, A. L., & Hall, N. R. Thymosin peptides and lymphokines do not directly stimulate adrenal corticosteroid production *in vitro*. *Journal of Immunology,* 1983, 130 (2), 791-794.

Vale, W., Rivier, C., Plotsky, P., Brown, M., Sawchenko, P., Bruhn, T., Seifert, H., Bilezikjian, L., Pandol, S., Perrin, M., Swanson, L., Fisher, L., Speiss, J., Thorner, M., & Rivier, J. Characterization of corticotropin and growth hormone releasing factors. In F. Labrie, & L. Proulx (Eds.), *International Congress of Endocrinology (7th: 1984: Québec, Québec)*. Amsterdam: Excerpta Medica, 1984.

van Epps, D. E., & Saland, L. β-Endorphin and met-enkephalin stimulate human peripheral blood mononuclear cell chemotaxis. *Journal of Immunology,* 1984, 132 (6), 3046-3053.

van Wimersma Greidanus, T. B., Bohus, B., Kovács, G. L., Versteeg, D. H. G., Burbach, J. P., & de Wied, D. Sites of behavioral and neurochemical action of ACTH-like peptides and neurohypophyseal hormones. *Neuroscience & Biobehavioral Reviews,* 1983, 7 (4), 453-463.

Williams, J. M., Peterson, R. G., Shea, P. A., Schmedtje, J. F., Bauer, D. C., & Felten, D. L. Sympathetic innervation of murine thymus and spleen: Evidence for a functional link between the nervous and immune systems. *Brain Research Bulletin,* 1981, 6 (1), 83-94.

Woloski, B. M., Smith, E. M., Meyer, W. J. 3d, Fuller, G. M., & Blalock, J. E. Corticotropin-releasing activity of monokines. *Science,* 1985, 230 (4729), 1035-1037.

Wybran, J., Appelboom, T., Famaey, J. P., & Govaerts, A. Suggestive evidence
    for receptors for morphine and methionine-enkephalin on normal human
    blood T lymphocytes. *Journal of Immunology,* 1979, 123 (3), 1068-1070.

Zaborszky, L. Afferent connections of the medial basal hypothalamus. *Advances in Anatomy, Embryology, and Cell Biology,* 1982, 69, 1-107.

Zukin, R. S., & Zukin, S. R. The case for multiple opiate receptors. *Trends in Neurosciences,* 1984, 7, 160-164.

Chapter 4

Immunity in Neuropsychiatric and Neurologic Illness

There are questions relating to the origin and outcome of disease that have a special poignancy when addressed to some of the more intransigent dilemmas in medicine. Is susceptibility to a given disease predetermined by inheritance? Alternatively, is it the consequence of environmental insult? Or must it be considered the consequence of both? Repeated almost to the point of banality, these questions nevertheless reflect the urgent, compassionate need to find the sorts of answers that can lead to effective forms of treatment: to break, for example, the "monolithic obstinacy" of schizophrenia (Himmelhoch, 1978), and to either ameliorate or cure the severe neurologic disorders that can debilitate so profoundly and pose a threat to life itself.

Immunology, neurology, psychiatry, and genetics merge today in this effort, with the result that more educated answers to these difficult questions are forthcoming at a more rapid pace than ever before. Immunology holds the key. As noted earlier, its technical sophistication has expanded enor-

77

mously the frontiers of neuroscience. Most importantly, the development of the hybridoma and specific antisera have given substance to the long held belief that one or another immune aberration may exist as corollary to phase change in neurologic and neuropsychiatric illness. As evidence of this advance, the technology required for the immunologic analysis, *per se*, of brain tissue, *post mortem*, and of cerebrospinal fluid (CSF) constitution, *in vivo*, is not only well in place, but sees continuous refinement. As further testimony to this advance, it is now possible, as part of an individualized treatment protocol, to target monoclonal antibodies to specific regulatory T cell subsets. Entire populations of lymphocytes that typically show deviation from optimum ratios in illnesses of this kind can now be equilibrated by this means (see, for example, Hafler et al., 1986).

Basic to whatever discoveries have yet to unfold in the immunologic study of these disorders—and there should be many—is the finding that immune components are capable of assailing the "privileged site" (Barker & Billingham, 1977) by breaching the blood-brain barrier (Goldstein & Betz, 1986). The extent of tissue damage that is presumed to result from this transudation into brain of plasma cells, antibody molecules, and T lymphocytes depends upon the disease in question, as well as upon the existing status of the disease, active (relapsed) or remitted, as the case may be.

It must be asked what single event or combination of events can have occurred to initiate this penetration. If the viral hypothesis may be said to be gaining a measure of acceptance, it is hardly on the strength of robust evidence to date. Tissue destruction, such as demyelination in multiple sclerosis (MS), no doubt occurs as sequel to serum protein leakage into brain through cerebral capillary cells, the initial destructive event. But is this influx through the intercellular junctions of capillary endothelia and interconnected astrocytes the consequence of local inflammatory response to invading virus? If so, why has it proven so difficult, if not impossible in most instances, to isolate an infectious agent? Where likely infectious viral agents abound, as in multiple sclerosis, why has it not been possible to demonstrate a causal connection? Also to be explained is the extensive, yet highly specific, undermining of neural tissue often seen in terminal stages of the diseases in question.

The following report is selective in its purpose and biased in its point of view. It is selective because it will solely emphasize three medical disorders involving the central nervous system: schizophrenia, systemic lupus erythematosus (SLE), and multiple sclerosis (MS). This choice is made on the grounds that, of the several that might be considered, these three are disorders on which a strong immunologic perspective has emerged. Also, despite their differences, these particular conditions exhibit like features that clinico-immunologic studies have helped to emphasize. Where they differ, it is interesting to speculate on *why* they differ. And if, at the present time, there should be no ready answer to this question, a kind of synthesis can be achieved by comparing what is presently known of immune abnormalities in (1) a psychiatric illness in which biochemical and morphologic abnormalities within the CNS are not an uncommon finding, (2) a systemic rheumatological disease with central, psychiatric involvement, and (3) a disease chiefly characterized by extensive demylinative lesions of the brain.

Medical research on the immunologic *versus* physiologic *versus* psychologic aspects of diseases in general has been anything but systematic, in the sense of having been consistently interdisciplinary. It is hardly surprising, therefore, that the development of an immunologic perspective on neuropsychiatric and neurologic disorders has been slow-paced and spasmodic. Immune abnormalities in schizophrenia have only recently become a focus of attention, a research bias that obviously reflects a preoccupation with the cardinal clinical features of the illness. With respect to systemic lupus erythematosus, the physiologic syndrome is, of itself, so protean as to have given its psychologic component an almost incidental aspect. In multiple sclerosis, the devastating impact of neuronal damage has been perceived as primarily physiologic, with the result that behavioral and emotional concomitants of the disease have remained virtually unexplored (Schiffer & Babigian, 1984; Schiffer & Slater, 1985).

This report is biased in the sense that we have chosen to concentrate on the concept of autoimmunity, as it might apply to any one of these three medical conditions. It is a concept that has undergone intermittent scrutiny, remains viable, yet controversial. Most interestingly, it is one of two recurrent themes in the research literature that may yet prove to be mutually inclusive, the other being the question of viral etiology.

With respect to schizophrenia, our selective approach is not in any way intended to controvert a literature that is preeminently psychodynamic in emphasis. Rather, our report on altered immune activity in schizophrenia will outline new research (some of it a confirmation of earlier work) that promises to offer a fresh look at its pathogenesis. To quote from a 1978 paper by Jonathan M. Himmelhoch: "it is not...a 'far-out' possibility that there are subgroups of schizophrenic reactions that have their roots in the immune system, and that present immuno-research is now sophisticated and elegant enough to begin pursuit of these will o' the wisps" (p. 26).

In fact, were immunologic profile analysis of the schizophrenias (Crow, 1981) to be undertaken on a broad scale, its outcome would be likely to have a considerable impact on the closely allied disciplines of psychopharmacology and psychotherapeutics (Goldstein et al., 1980). Not the least stimulus to a general reappraisal of treatment regimens, alone, would come of the discovery that antipsychotic drugs, including the neuroleptic drug, chlorpromazine (CPZ), are detrimental to normal immune function (Goldstein et al., 1980). Chlorpromazine has been shown to decrease the total number and percentage of T lymphocytes (Nyland, Naess, & Lunde, 1980), to be associated with leukocyte abnormalities (Fieve, Blumenthal, & Little, 1966), and to induce the formation of antinuclear antibodies (Alarçon-Segovia et al., 1973; Zarrabi et al., 1979).

Mental and emotional disturbances are considered adjunctive features of systemic lupus erythematosus. It is noteworthy, however, that just such features tend to correlate with heightened immune reactivity. In its most florid phase, this prototypic autoimmune disease can manifest symptoms similar to schizophrenia: e.g., visual and auditory hallucinations, paranoia, extreme withdrawal, etc. (Carr et al., 1978). It is indeed a striking illustration of the close links between psyche, soma, and immunity when it can be shown that chlorpromazine therapy will induce *physical* symptoms very like lupus in *psychotic* patients, including the appearance of antinuclear antibodies (Ananth & Mihn, 1973; Dubois, Tallman, & Wonka, 1972).

Finally, there is the pervasive question of vulnerability. To what extent does genetic makeup predispose the individual to these serious health hazards? That there is a genetic basis for predisposition to various chronic diseases, including a number of autoimmune disorders, is now an accepted fact (Ryder, Platz, & Svejgaard, 1981). The typing of tissue antigens defined by the histocompatibility gene complex, or HLA system (Dick & Kissmeyer-Nielsen, 1979), has led to the identification of genetic markers for multiple sclerosis (Jersild, 1978), systemic lupus erythematosus (Ravech, 1984; Walport et al., 1982), and schizophrenia (Gottesman & Shields, 1972, 1976).

Questions remain, however. With regard to schizophrenia, the search for genetic linkage has met with less than stunning success, owing in large part to the fact that schizophrenia, like multiple sclerosis and SLE, does not represent a single disease entity. For *process* schizophrenia, where there is a family history of endogenous psychosis, HLA associations have been reported (Fessel, Hirata-Hibi, & Shapiro, 1965). So, too, for paranoid and hebephrenic subtypes, and schizophrenic twins (Kinney & Matthysse, 1978; Nurnberger & Gershon, 1982). However, no particular haplotype has yet been identified (Rosler et al., 1983). Neither linkage, nor consistent association of HLA antigens with any one of the pathophysiologic deficits in schizophrenia hve been convincingly demonstrated. Finally, it has not been possible to establish an unambiguous connection between apparent HLA associations and genetic transmission of the illness (Gershon & Nurnberger, 1982).

There is not solid enough evidence to classify any portion of the "spectrum of schizophrenia" (Bleuler, 1911; Reich, 1975) as an autoimmune disorder (Möller, 1983), and it is by no means certain that immune abnormalities in schizophrenia necessarily play a role in its pathogenesis. These uncertainties notwithstanding, there are a number of immunologic disturbances in schizophrenia that point to autoimmunity. Also, certain similarities can be drawn between schizophrenia and those neurologic diseases that show frank autoimmune features. Our discussion opens, therefore, with a review of the kinds of data that continue to support this enduring thesis.

IMMUNE ABNORMALITIES IN SCHIZOPHRENIA

Humoral Immunity

In 1912, V.K. Khorshkho suggested that neuropsychiatric disorders were as much a manifestation of immunologic, as of psychologic, derangement and quite evidently viewed autoimmunity (so very young a concept at the time!) as an entirely plausible explanation for certain of the manifestations of psychiatric illness. Revived in the late 1930s (Lehmann-Facius, 1939), and again in the early 1960s (Fessel, 1962, 1963; Kouzhetzova & Seminov, 1961), the autoimmune hypothesis of schizophrenia has been largely based on evidence that globulin-like substances, obtained both from the sera of schizophrenic patients, as well as from the brains of such patients at time of autopsy, bind to brain tissue with marked affinity, as compared to like specimens obtained from normal individuals (see De-Lisi, Weber, & Pert, 1985; Janković, 1985a; Solomon, 1981, for recent reviews).

Whatever their role in the pathogenesis of schizophrenia, the presence of these potentially autoreactive agents in sera of a percentage of normal individuals obviously disqualifies them as "markers" for schizophrenia. Even the oligodendroglial-specific serum globulin fraction, taraxein, first thought to be specific to schizophrenia (Heath & Krupp, 1967), has been detected in normal sera (Bergen et al., 1980). Furthermore, antineuronal antibodies are commonly found in serum in multiple sclerosis (Ryberg, 1982; Trotter & Brooks, 1980) and systemic lupus erythematosus (Bluestein & Zvaifler, 1976).

It has been proposed that autoreactive molecules observed in schizophrenia, or so-called antibrain antibodies (Janković, 1972), may target autologous receptor structures in the CNS, and as either agonists or antagonists to transmitters, mimic or block normal neurosecretory activity, with profound consequences to mental and emotional equilibrium (DeLisi et al., 1985; Fudenberg et al., 1983; Knight, 1982, 1984). This premise—namely, that receptor for transmitter may function as antigen—derives directly from the proven immunopathologic mediation of neuromuscular blockage in the autoimmune disease, myasthenia gravis, where antibody is known to act against the acetylcholine receptor in muscle (Carnegie & Mackay, 1975; Lindstrom et al., 1976; Patrick & Lindstrom, 1973). If proven applicable to schizophrenia, this idea might help to explain the increased concentrations of norepinephrine (Farley et al., 1978) and its precursor, dopamine (Crow, 1981), found in the mesolimbic structures of schizophrenic brain, *post mortem*.

Branislav D. Janković and his group have led the way in analyzing the biological activity of these antibrain molecules, *in vivo*, reporting electroencephalographic disturbances in a number of different animal models following the intraventricular injection of antibody (Janković, 1972). They have also recorded the effects of antibrain immunoglobulins on the evoked action potential, spike activity, resistance, capacitance, etc., of neurons, *in vitro* (Janković, 1985a).

By inference, alterations of this kind might be expected to be reflected in behavior. Just such supportive evidence in fact antedated the neurophysiologic findings. In experiments performed in the 1960s, Janković's group showed that antibrain antibodies "profoundly affected" both electroencephalographic activity and conditioned behavior when injected intraventricularly in cats (Janković et al., 1968; Mihailović & Janković, 1961; Mihailović et al., 1969). Later work has replicated these early results, confirming the detrimental effects of antibrain globulin on behavior, learning and memory processes (see Janković, 1985a, for review).

At this juncture, further technical and procedural refinements are essential in order that issues surrounding these potentially significant findings can be clarified. To paraphrase a statement to this effect by Lynn E. DeLisi and colleagues (1985): antibody detection assays must be optimized, and the biochemistry of individual brain binding antibodies characterized; new technology must be applied to the visualization of regional CNS distribution patterns of those antigens recognized by antibodies from individual schizophrenic patients; and finally, the phenomenon of antibrain antibody binding to brain tissue from schizophrenic patients, a finding from earlier studies (Heath & Krupp, 1967; Lehmann-Facius, 1939), deserves further investigation.

Although the literature on the topic is anything but concordant, it is apparent that the schizophrenias show peripheral, as well as central, abnormalities in humoral immunity that are indicative of autoreactivity. Over the past 30 years, there have been reports of elevated versus decreased serum and CSF immunoglobulin levels (IgA, IgG, IgM) in acute *versus* chronic, medicated *versus* unmedicated, male *versus* female, black *versus* white schizophrenic patients. Correlations have been noted between these immune abnormalities, severity of symptoms, and subgroup classification (see Solomon, 1981, for review).

Parallels have also been drawn between schizophrenia and the auto-immune disorders, rheumatoid arthritis and systemic lupus erythematosus, on the grounds that all three conditions show serum immunoglobulin elevation, notably IgA and IgM—an argument that has been thought tenuous, at best (Weiner, 1985). In his recent overview of this particular research area—writing, moreover, as one of its pioneers—George F. Solomon (1981) offered the following comment, that, if not optimistic, may well be appropriate to a still-developing field: "Although theoretically attractive for its potential to integrate genetic and stress factors, the work on schizophrenia as a specific autoimmune disease, with antibrain an-tibodies playing a pathogenic role, is not convincing" (p. 273).

Cell-Mediated Immunity

Studies that have evaluated T cell-mediated responsiveness in schiz-ophrenia suggest that cellular processes may also contribute importantly to its symptomatology. The Janković group has demonstrated positive delayed skin hypersensitivity to two nonencephalitogenic constituent proteins of neuron-glial complexes, i.e., human brain S-100 protein and neuron-specific enolase (NSE), in the majority of their schizophrenic patient sample (Janković, 1985b; Janković, Jakulić, & Horvat, 1980, 1982). Once again, it should be noted that this sensitivity was not patho-gnomonic for schizophrenia, inasmuch as positive reactions were obtained from a small percentage of normal control subjects, as well as from other individuals in the total patient pool (N=1010) suffering from a variety of disorders (i.e., dementia, depression, cerebral atrophy of unknown origin, mental retardation and alcoholism). In addition, Janković (1985b) has pointed to the possible confounding effect of antipsychotic drug treatment on the skin hypersensitivity response (no one of the schizophrenic group was drug-free).

Most recently, Janković (1985b) has suggested that because S-100 protein is associated with pigmented neuromelanin-containing cells in the dorsal substantia nigra of the mesencephalon, cells that also contain the neurotransmitter, dopamine, the protein might play some part in the dis-turbances of transmitter synthesis and uptake that are thought to affect this particular neuronal network in some forms of schizophrenia (Crow, 1981; Meltzer & Stahl, 1976).

As closing comment on immunity and schizophrenia, a 1985 study that may have identified a basis for discrimination between schizophrenia and major depressive disorder deserves special mention. Steven J. Schleifer and coworkers (1985) have reported that, whereas drug-free schizophrenic patients (N=16) were not found to differ immunologically from healthy age- and sex-matched control subjects on the basis of either T and B lymphocyte number, or stimulation response to mitogen, ambulatory patients (N=15) with acute depressive disorder showed a significant decrease in absolute number of T cells as compared to a separate control group, mitogen-induced lymphocyte stimulation response showing no difference between groups in this latter comparison.

IMMUNE ABNORMALITIES IN SYSTEMIC LUPUS ERYTHEMATOSUS

Humoral Immunity

To arrive at a correct initial diagnosis of systemic lupus erythematosus can be a difficult clinical task. For one thing, the disease can present with symptoms of multiple sclerosis (Allan et al., 1979; Fulford et al., 1972). For another, its two generally contrasting symptom clusters, systemic and cerebral, show degrees of dissociation. That is to say, there may be little or no sign of the polyarthritis and pervasive vasculitis indicative of systemic involvement even as CNS damage is taking place (Ellis & Verity, 1979; Richardson, 1980). Not surprisingly, in a literature that is rife with contradiction, there are also reports of positive, unambiguous association between the two forms of the disease (Feinglass et al., 1976).

These unstable disease attributes have been subjected to lengthy analysis and are of obvious importance to diagnostics. However, our attention is better directed to that form of systemic lupus erythematosus involving the central nervous system primarily, hence remarkable for its associated disturbances in cognitive function and behavior.

Firstly, fluctuations in antineuronal immunoglobulin activity in the active disease phase tend to be correlated with neuropsychiatric dysfunction (Carr et al., 1978; Swaak et al., 1982). Secondly, elevations in the ratio of immunoglobulin G to total protein in cerebrospinal fluid (CSF) in CNS lupus eythematosus are directly correlated with injury to the choroid plexus, this plexus being the circumventricular capillary structure that comprises the blood-CSF barrier.

Breaching of the Blood-CSF Barrier

Two pathological events are thought to contribute to pleocytosis (excess of leukocytes) in cerebrospinal fluid and immune cell penetration of the choroid plexus in CNS lupus erythematosus. The first is *de novo* synthesis of antibody in brain and cerebrospinal fluid. The second is a local inflammatory reaction to the deposition of gamma globulin and DNA:anti-DNA immune complexes at the junction of choroid basement membrane and epithelial cells surrounding capillary plexi within the membrane (see Carr et al., 1978, for review).

It has not escaped notice that obvious parallels exist between two of the more striking physiologic manifestations of lupus erythematosus. It is presumed that two otherwise disparate tissue loci, the brain choroid plexus and the juxtaglomerular apparatus of the kidney, are injured by similar mechanisms, given their similarity of function and ultrastructural composition. Each operates as a large filter capable of protein entrapment (Brightman, 1975; Brightman, Zis, & Anders, 1983; McIntosh et al., 1973). This property alone could account for the autoreactive subversion of choroid capillary matrices by immunoglobulin, quite as it apparently contributes to glomerular basement membrane injury in SLE glomerulonephritis (McIntosh & Koss, 1974). A still more convincing parallel stems from the 1973 discovery by R.M. McIntosh and colleagues that choroid plexus and glomerular basement membranes share antigenic characteristics.

Antineuronal Antibodies and Neuropsychiatric Dysfunction

The presence of neurocytotoxic antibody—or, stated more precisely, autoantibody bound to nuclear deoxyribonucleoprotein (DNA-protein)—is considered a hallmark of CNS lupus erythematosus (as observed by indirect immunofluorescence and the measurement of anti-DNA antibody "avidity" [Farr radioimmunoassay]) (Russell, 1981). Two other signs distinguishing cerebral from systemic (principally renal) involvement in the disease are: (1) evidence in serum of antibodies to neuronal membrane antigens (Bluestein, 1984); and (2) the presence of cytotoxic antibodies that cross-react with antigenic determinants on T lymphocytes and human brain tissue (Bluestein & Zvaifler, 1976; Charlesworth, Quin, & Yasmeen, 1983). Which of these two types of antibody correlates more exactly with the neuropsychiatric aspects of lupus is not yet determined. Also, as Bluestein (1984) has recently noted, a still more fundamental question remains unanswered: what might be "the nature of the antigenic stimulus inducing the antineuronal activity" (p. 163)?

This correlation between autoantibody reactivity to nuclear and cytoplasmic elements of central neurons and onset of schizophrenic-like disturbance in CNS lupus is reminiscent of the connection between antibody-mediated reactivity to brain tissue, and its evident consequences to mentation and emotion, in schizophrenia itself. In fact, to Ronald I. Carr and colleagues (1978), the often coincidental occurrence of immune aberrance, brain pathophysiology, and psychologic dysfunction seen in CNS lupus strongly implies that a cluster of similar pathologic processes might contribute to schizophrenia. It is worthy of note that these authors draw such parallels between the two disorders in a paper that includes for review the several lines of evidence that suggest a viral origin for systemic lupus erythematosus.

IMMUNE ABNORMALITIES IN MULTIPLE SCLEROSIS

Humoral and Cellular Immunity

A 1984 paper on immunologic abnormalities in neurologic disease, including multiple sclerosis (MS), concludes with the statement: "it is painfully obvious that the etiology and pathogenesis of MS are not known" (McFarlin, 1984, p. 243). It is a statement that could as well describe the disconcertment experienced by investigators involved in schizophrenia and SLE research.

Seen from the perspective of a general overview, these separate fields of investigation would seem not only to be cataloguing some of the same, or similar, phenomena, but also to be developing the same, or similar, interpretive arguments to account for them. Thus, patients with multiple sclerosis, like those with systemic lupus erythematosus and schizophrenia, show evidence of immunoglobulins in cerebrospinal fluid. In addition, although the presence of antibody to myelin basic protein in cerebrospinal fluid (not serum) is a generally reliable barometer of multiple sclerosis in exacerbation, it, like antibrain antibody in schizophrenia, is not specific to the disease (Bashir & Whitaker, 1980).

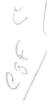

Again, whereas the percentage of MS patients with elevated autoantibody titer is typically high (Johnson, 1980; Link et al., 1977), patients are apt to present with such individual variation in CSF immunoglobulin titer as to disqualify this particular parameter as a diagnostic criterion for the disease. Again, too, the conviction grows with respect to multiple sclerosis, as to schizophrenia and CNS lupus, that an abnormal spinal fluid protein content is indicative of synthesis *de novo*: in other words, immunoglobulin synthesis and immune complex production within the spinal cord and brain (Tourtellotte et al., 1980).

Multiple sclerosis or, to use its more exact descriptive label, sclerosing encephalomyelitis, is classified as an organ-specific, autoallergic disease (Gottlieb, 1970). It is also a disease for which there has been no want of hypotheses concerning etiology and pathogenesis, the viral hypothesis of etiology having remained firm.

It is not the least remarkable that the idea of a viral etiology persists. There have been estimated to be as many as 10^8 B cell-derived plasma cells (antibody-producing cells) sequestered in the perivascular compartments of the brain in patients with multiple sclerosis (Prineas & Wright, 1978). What, it has been asked, is the antigenic target for the bulk of antibody, aside from the "small portion" known to be directed either against myelin or against the viral proteins so commonly detected in MS patients, such as rubella, herpes simplex, measles, etc. (Whitaker, 1984)? Or, as Arnason, Antel, and Reder (1984) have pointedly observed: "a substantial proportion of patients have antibodies to several viruses at the same time. Although it could be argued that any given virus might be the cause of MS, they cannot all be" (p. 137). Yet, it is thought that until an exogenous source of CNS infection specific to the disease is identified, one against which either antibody or cell-mediated hypersensitivity can be demonstrated, it will prove difficult to arrive at any firm conclusions with respect to viral cause and/or autoimmune mediation in multiple sclerosis (Lisak et al., 1984).

The search for the identity of an infectious agent has of course provided a driving force to basic research on the origins of the disease. The search has gained equally in sharper focus and greater breadth with the passage of time and technological advance, for it has had to take into account both the mechanisms of autoimmunity, as these are presently (and imperfectly) understood, as well as the sometimes perplexing repercussions of immune system response to what is generally agreed to be a disease-precipitating assault by virus.

The search has been disappointing. It would in fact be an understatement to say that the evident absence of disease-specific antigen in MS, coupled with the all-too-obvious persistence of a sensitivity response, despite its absence, has presented researchers in the field with a conundrum—not to mention a basis for wide-ranging speculation. However, because interpretation of the enigma is more generally relevant to the subject matter of this chapter as a whole, and relates, in a quite specific way, to an aspect of our foregoing review of immune system function, *per se*, we will delay until our summary remarks further consideration of antigenic specificity relative to invasive immunogen(s).

The Break in Self Tolerance

For the present, we turn to the subject of self antigen in what is nominally an autoimmune disorder of marked specificity. There is, first of all, the "given:" myelin basic protein (MBP), a principal protein-lipid constituent of the fatty sheath surrounding neurons (Norton, 1981), is proven to induce encephalitis. Although yet to be demonstrated in humans, this cell-mediated hypersensitivity reaction has long been under study in the condition known as experimental allergic encephalomyelitis (EAE), an analogue for demyelinating neurologic disease developed in susceptible animals by peripheral inoculation of myelin base protein or MBP peptide constituents: as for example, the ganglioside, galactocerebroside (GalC) (Hashim, 1978; Kolb, 1950; Waksman, 1959).

Inflammatory, immunologically-mediated demyelination signifies the presence of self antigens specific either to myelin itself or to the glial cells that produce and maintain the myelin sheath, i.e., oligodendrocytes in brain and Schwann cells of the peripheral nervous system (PNS) (Lisak, 1984). But for some few exceptions, including human MBP, the mapping of the entire 169-amino acid myelin basic protein molecule is now complete (Braun & Brostoff, 1977; Carnegie & Dunkley, 1975). Its ten-amino acid "encephalitogenic site" also has been defined, showing an antigenic profile that is species-specific (Shapira et al., 1971).

What are the antigenic characteristics of myelin and its associated glia? And is there but one autoantigen responsible for demyelination? Apparently not. Demyelination will occur following exposure of galactocerebroside (GalC) to mouse monoclonal Ig M antibody, *in vitro*, indicating that there may exist more than a single vulnerable locus or self determinant on the myelin molecule to account for its antigenicity. Whether GalC acts as an autoantigen in multiple sclerosis, as well as in EAE, has not been determined. There is some question also as to whether the oligodendrocyte, rather then myelin, might not function as primary, initiating tissue target in disease onset (Lisak, 1984; Lisak et al., 1984).

In view of the fact that the EAE model is applicable to demyelinating neurologic disorders in general, and not to MS specifically, there is a less-than-perfect concordance between the two conditions. Myelin-specific sera immunoglobulin (IgG, IgM) from animals with experimental allergic encephalitis and from patients with multiple sclerosis both show demyelinating reactivity to rodent CNS tissue, in culture (Bornstein, & Appel, 1965). Yet, later studies undertaken to replicate and expand upon this early finding have yielded contradictory results (see Lisak et al., 1984, for review).

Immune Cell Interactions in Multiple Sclerosis

Changes in the migratory pattern and localization of immunocompetent cells, as well as changes in their relative proportions and absolute numbers, are symptomatic of multiple sclerosis, being closely associated with periods of disease exacerbation and remission (Cashman et al., 1982; Sandberg-Wollhein, 1983). Moreover, different classes of cells, including phagocytic cells (macrophages), natural killer (NK) cells, antibody-producing plasma cells, and various T cell subsets, appear either to be actively involved in, or in some way affected by, the ongoing disease process. Not fully understood are: (1) the respective contributions of these different cell types to the destructive CNS demyelinative lesions, or plaques, characteristic of MS; and (2) the temporal relationship between such formation and immune reactivity, as reflected in cerebrospinal fluid, brain specimen, and serum analyses. To quote from a 1984 paper by Lisak and colleagues: "even if antibodies to myelin are found in the sera and CSF of patients with MS, it may be a consequence of demyelination rather than a cause" (p. 222).

Macrophage aggregation at the site of CNS lesions is a typical, but unexplained, finding in multiple sclerosis. In evident reflection of macrophage activity, specimens of myelin base protein, or peptide fragments thereof, have been isolated from the cerebrospinal fluid of patients with active MS, these being the presumed degradation products of proteinases secreted by stimulated macrophages circulating both in brain and cerebrospinal fluid (Cammer et al., 1978). As tissue debris, it is not unlikely that such fragments constitute antigenic material that must then stimulate still further immunologic response, so perpetuating the auto-aggressive cycle.

There is new evidence to show that macrophages may be responsible for an episodic immunologic imbalance that is synchronous with the cyclical nature of this progressive disease. A comprehensive study, undertaken in 1984 by Merrill, Myers, and Ellison, has confirmed the work of others in finding a reduction in the responsiveness of natural killer (NK) cells in multiple sclerosis, relative to schizophenia and other neurologic diseases, as measured by the ^{51}Cr-release assay, a test of NK cell killing, recycling, and rekilling efficacy (Ullberg & Jondal, 1981). (Reduced numbers of NK cells were found only in acute MS patients.)

The authors attributed the reduction in NK cell activity to the inhibiting effect of prostaglandins (PGE) released by activated macrophages, citing the well known inhibitory effect of these potent aliphatic acids on immune cell cytotoxicity through their stimulation of intracellular concentrations of cyclic AMP. Abnormally elevated levels of prostaglandin were also found in the spinal fluid of the MS patient group. In view of the fact that these PGE levels neither correlated with total count, nor percentage, of phagocytes in the fluid, they were judged to result from the secretory activity of macrophages within the central nervous system. Another significant observation was that NK cells taken from peripheral blood in the multiple sclerosis patients showed increased sensitivity to prostaglandin, in contrast to cell samples taken from control subjects. Not unexpectedly, study of the effect of prostaglandin on NK cell surface receptor number, sensitivity, affinity, and turnover is a projected next step in this research.

It is also of interest that Merrill and his group found K (killer) cell activity against antibody-coated target cells, *in vitro* (the so-called antibody-dependent cell-mediated cytotoxicity [ADCC] response), to be elevated in the MS group. This elevation probably results from the fact that, in contrast to NK cytotoxicity, K cell cytotoxicity is an immune parameter that is relatively insensitive to prostaglandin influence ("NK effectors are sensitive to PGE1 at a 100-fold lower concentration than their ADCC-effector counterparts" [Merrill et al., 1984, p. 199]).

The noted imbalance is a telling abnormality on three counts. In the first place, NK cell activity and antibody-dependent cell-mediated cytotoxicity normally exist in equilibrium. In the second place, disequilibrium between the two functions may help to distinguish between relapsing/remitting *versus* chronic/progressive forms of multiple sclerosis. In the third place, the disequilibrium may prove to be an identifying marker for the disease, it having been lacking in all other individuals tested in this study.

Under normal circumstances in healthy individuals, populations of regulatory T helper (T_4) and T suppressor/cytotoxic ($T_5/_8$) cells show moderate fluctuation around an optimum, if disproportionate, ratio (usually less than 4), T_4 cells constituting approximately 65 per cent of the total T cell population. However, in relapsing/remitting multiple sclerosis, this ratio fluctuates far more radically, showing a T_4/T_8 ratio of 5 or more at times of acute disease activity and a return to more nearly normal ratios occurring during disease quiescence (Reder et al., 1984; Weiner & Hauser, 1982). An increased T_4/T_8 ratio is not, of itself, a diagnostic tool, being an abnormality of immunoregulation that is symptomatic of hyper- or autoimmune activity—it is seen in systemic lupus erythematosus (Morimoto et al., 1980)—but has proven a useful index of disease severity (Antel, Arnason, & Medof, 1979; Hauser et al., 1983b) and a guide to treatment (Hauser et al., 1982).

It is also a puzzling finding for which there is no certain explanation. It has been proposed that the disturbance may be the consequence of suppressor T cell—and to a more limited extent, helper T cell—sequestration in the central nervous system (Traugott, Stone, & Raine, 1978; Weiner et al., 1984b). The idea is plausible, given the noted changes in peripheral T cell concentrations, combined with immunohistological evidence of T_8 cell excess relative to T_4 cells in plaques in autopsied MS brain tissue (Booss et al., 1983; Traugott, Reinherz, & Raine, 1983; Weiner et al., 1984a).

Immune and Brain Cell Interactions in Multiple Sclerosis

However preliminary, these findings have sufficed to introduce the next area of inquiry. How else to account for the infiltration of lymphocytes into brain other than to infer the presence in brain of specific stimuli capable of diverting these cells from their usual patterns of movement in systemic compartments?

If one were to take into account the fact that macrophages, and a small percentage of microglia, clustered at CNS lesion sites display Ia-positive surface antigens (Hauser et al., 1983a; Weiner et al., 1984a), a possible rationale for activated T cell traffic from periphery to brain might suggest itself. Astrocytes are coming to be considered primary "facultative, inducible" antigen-presenting cells within the central nervous system (Wekerle et al., 1986). Furthermore, it is conceivable that macrophages, drawn to brain parenchyma by mechanisms yet unknown, might, in combination with resident Ia-bearing glial cells, significantly alter immune cell dynamics.

The validity of this idea depends upon whether similar kinds of attractant forces operate in and between both tissue spheres, central and peripheral (Hauser & Weiner, 1984). The Ia (immune response-associated) antigen figures importantly in the sequential precision process by which T cells become activated. It will be remembered that in order to effect T cell maturation, proliferation, and reactivity, certain restrictive criteria must be met: the histocompatibility molecule must be presented in sufficient density; its molecular profile must be recognized *in conjunction* with that of the foreign antigen; and the presentation must be accompanied by release of stimulatory monokines by an accessory cell, such as the macrophage (Schwartz, Yano, & Paul, 1978).

There is preliminary evidence that circulating peripheral lymphocytes may indeed be influenced by MHC-restriction signals received from non-neuronal cells within the brain. In a 1984 paper, Fontana, Fierz, and Wekerle reported the induction of surface Ia antigen on cultured, primed astrocytes to be a function of "specific contact" with an MBP-specific, i.e., encephalitogenic, T cell line, whereas Ia expression in cultured, naive astrocytes was not demonstrable.

Then too, the possibility cannot be overlooked that brain matter might *itself* affect lymphocyte activity. Endogenous ganglioside, the glycosphin-golipid constituent of myelin base protein, has been shown capable of stimulating thymocyte proliferation (Speigel et al., 1984, 1985).

Given what we know of influence and counter-influence in bodily processes involving the immune system, it is perhaps to be expected that a factor (lymphokine?) obtained from the supernatant of mitogen-stimulated T cells would have been found to induce neuroglial cell proliferation, *in vitro* (Fontana et al., 1980). This finding has been corroborated, *in vivo*, by an experiment demonstrating that proliferation of glia in rat brain can be blocked (in a manner, and by a route, as yet undefined) by pretreatment of the animal with the immunosuppressive drug, methotrexate (MTX), prior to mechanically-induced trauma to the frontal cortex (Billingsley, Hall, & Mandel, 1982).

This type of lesion typically gives rise to a proliferative response in astroglia (Kitamura, 1980), preliminary to plaque formation. But that the response may not be solely T cell-mediated is indicated by the report of Giulian and Lachman (1985) showing astrocyte proliferation following brain trauma to be stimulated by interleukin 1 (IL-1). The source of the monokine—whether from invading or resident mononuclear cell—remains undetermined.

CONCLUSIONS

Today, it is in the power of molecular biology to give substance to phantoms in medicine. Computer-assisted amino acid sequence analysis and the monoclonal antibody probe are but two of a new class of precision tools that promise to dispel a number of mysteries surrounding the origins of certain diseases. One such mystery has been highlighted in this chapter by our having looked at three medical syndromes from the narrow point of view of immunology. We have noted, in each case, the signs of a protracted immunologic response—but to a phantom antigen.

We conclude this chapter with an example of the manner in which esoteric problems of this sort are being approached in the laboratory. This single example also tells us the extent to which ongoing research is compatible with a theoretical framework that stands as a triumph of modern immunology: the concept of idiotypy as vehicle for immune regulation.

The encephalitogenic site of rabbit myelin base protein and hepatitis B virus polymerase (HBVP) share an homologous sequence of amino acids.

This homology consists of just six amino acids in linear sequence. Yet, antibody raised in rabbit against the appropriate amino acid HBVP peptide fragment also reacts against the self-epitope on myelin.

In two steps, Fujinami and Oldstone (1985) have provided a classic illustration of antibody cross-reactivity to both self and foreign epitope moieties. They have then extrapolated from this finding to argue for the concept of molecular mimicry. To quote: "virus and host determinants must be sufficiently similar to induce a cross-reactive response, but different enough to break tolerance" (p. 1045). In "hit and run" fashion, the immunogen need only provoke the immune system into an autoallergic response before giving every indication of having vanished. By this subterfuge, it will have found asylum, and commandeered the means to its own survival, by having gained access to intracellular compartments in host tissue.

As we know, idiotypes and the idiotypic network affect stringent control over self-reactive lymphocyte clones (Jerne, 1974). To use the phrase "molecular mimicry" is to describe a circumstance in which subtle subversion of this regulatory system has taken place. In this circumstance, idiotype must represent a quasiimmunogen at best, one that may, or may not, be capable of stimulating antiidiotypic antibodies into production.

An alternative view of the strategem of mimicry, suggested by Janice R. Stevens (1982) in a recent editorial on the neuropathology of schizophrenia, is that, in yet another opportunistic guise, virus itself may compete with *neurotransmitter* "for the same, or closely related, binding sites on neural membrane," and so contribute to transmitter uptake blockade (p. 698). It is an alternative view that does not exclude the possibility of cross-reactivity.

Is any one, or are all, of the three medical disorders described in this chapter virally-induced? Is any one, or are they all, disorders of autoimmunity? It is not to be doubted that there are arguments to be mounted on both sides of both questions. Nor is it in doubt that documented evidence in support of such arguments is of such scope as to be far beyond the scope of this review.

We have cited the Fujinami and Oldstone study on the immune consequences of chemical homology between host and viral proteins not simply because it is provocative, but because it essentially annuls the issue. Schizophrenia, systemic (CNS) lupus erythematosus, and multiple sclerosis may each be correctly viewed as an autoimmune disorder that is viral in etiology.

We have also laid emphasis on a single neuropathologic aspect of multiple sclerosis, namely, glial scarring, because it helps to illustrate, in microcosm, the inseparableness of systems. Thus, first evidence would have it appear that by their presentation of immunogenic material in association with self-Ia glycoprotein, as well by as their release of interleukin 1, glial cells are able to activate and recruit T effector lymphocytes, whose signal molecules then stimulate the proliferation of glia.

The sequence seems in no way exceptional. Yet, it deserves a second look. Glial cells (i.e., astrocytes, oligodendrocytes, and the less differentiated microglials) comprise the most populous group of cells in the brain. Greatly outnumbering neurons (the relative proportion being something on the order of 10 to 1), glial cells are described as supportive, nutritive bodies juxtaposed between, and contiguous to, neurons and cerebral capillaries (Kandel, 1985). The fact that these cells can phagocytose, i.e., fulfill a scavenger role, in brain is well-known. But the fact that the neuroglia can also, in the strictest sense, behave as an accessory cell of the immune system is new information. To judge its full implication, one need only recall that the neuroglia is also an excitable cell (Abbott, 1985).

These first reports on immune responses within the central nervous system obscure the boundary zone between systems. Anomalies are being brought to light that must obviously challenge the interpretive resources of immunologist and neuroscientist alike. Apart from their theoretical import to psychoneuroimmunology, immunology, and neural science, it is inevitable that these discoveries will aid in the diagnosis and treatment of neuropsychiatric and neurologic illnesses.

REFERENCES

Abbott, N. J. Are glial cells excitable after all? *Trends in Neurosciences,* 1985, 8 (4), 141-142.

Alarcón-Segovia, D., Fishbein, E., Cetina, J. A., Raya, R. J., & Barrera, E. Antigenic specificity of chlorpromazine-induced antinuclear antibodies. *Clinical and Experimental Immunology,* 1973, 15 (4), 543-548.

Allen, I. V., Millar, J. H., Kirk, J., & Shillington, R. K. Systemic lupus erythematosus clinically resembling multiple sclerosis and with unusual pathological and ultrastructural features. *Journal of Neurology, Neurosurgery, and Psychiatry,* 1979, 42 (5), 392-401.

Ananth, J. V., & Minn, K. Chlorpromazine-induced systemic lupus erythematosus. *Canadian Medical Association Journal,* 1973, 108 (6), 680.

Antel, J. P., Arnason, B. G., & Medof, M. E. Suppressor cell function in multiple sclerosis: Correlation with clinical disease activity. *Annals of Neurology,* 1979, 5 (4), 338-342.

Arnason, B. G., Antel, J. P., & Reder, A. T. Immunoregulation in multiple sclerosis. *Annals of the New York Academy of Sciences,* 1984, 436, 133-139.

Barker, C. F., & Billingham, R. E. Immunologically privileged sites. *Advances in Immunology,* 1977, 25,1-54.

Bashir, R. M., & Whitaker, J. N. Molecular features of immunoreactive myelin basic protein in cerebrospinal fluid of persons with multiple sclerosis. *Annals of Neurology,* 1980, 7 (1), 50-57.

Bergen, J. R., Grinspoon, L., Pyle, H. M., Martinez, J. L., Jr., & Pennell, R. B. Immunologic studies in schizophrenic and control subjects. *Biological Psychiatry,* 1980, 15 (3), 369-379.

Billingsley, M. L., Hall, N., & Mandel, H. G. Trauma-induced glial proliferation: Possible involvement of the immune system. *Immunopharmacology,* 1982, 5 (2), 95-101.

Bleuler, E. Dementia praecox, oder die Gruppe der Schizophrenien. In G. Aschaffenburg (Ed.), *Handbuch der Psychiatrie.* Leipzig: F. Deuticke, 1911. (English translation, 1950)

Bluestein, H. G. Antineuronal antibodies in the pathogenesis of neuropsychiatric manifestations of systemic lupus erythematosus. In P. O. Behan & F. Spreafico (Eds.), *Neuroimmunology.* (Serono Sympiosia publications from Raven Press, Vol. 12.) New York: Raven Press, 1984, 157-165.

Bluestein, H. G., & Zvaifler, N. J. Brain-reactive lymphocytotoxic antibodies in the serum of patients with systemic lupus erythematosus. *Journal of Clinical Investigation,* 1976, 57 (2), 509-516.

Booss, J., Esiri, M. M., Tourtellotte, W. W., & Mason, D. Y. Immunohistological analysis of T lymphocyte subsets in the central nervous sytem in chronic progressive multiple sclerosis. *Journal of Neurology Science,* 1983, 62 (1-3), 219-232.

Bornstein, M. B., & Appel, S. A. Tissue culture studies of demyelination. *Annals of the New York Academy of Sciences,* 1965, 122, 280-286.

Braun, P. E., & Brostoff, S. W. Proteins of myelin. In P. Morrell (Ed.), *Myelin.* New York: Plenum Press, 1977, 201-231.

Brightman, M. W. Ultrastructural characteristics of adult choroid plexus: Relation to the blood-cerebrospinal fluid barrier to proteins. In M. G. Netsky & S. Shuangshoti (Eds.), *The Choroid Plexus in Health and Disease.* Charlottesville: University of Virginia Press, 1975, 86-112.

Brightman, M. W., Zis, K., & Anders, J. Morphology of cerebral endothelium and astrocytes as determinants of the neuronal microenvironment. *Acta Neuropathologica [Suppl.]* (Berlin), 1983, 8, 21-33.

Cammer, W., Bloom, B. R., Norton, W. T., & Gordon, S. Degradation of basic protein in myelin by neutral proteases secreted by stimulated macrophages: A possible mechanism of inflammatory demyelination. *Proceedings of the National Academy of Sciences, U.S.A.,* 1978, 75 (3), 1554-1558.

Carnegie, P. R., & Dunkley, P. R. Basic proteins of central and peripheral nervous system myelin. *Advances in Neurochemistry,* 1975, 1, 96-135.

Carnegie, P. R., & Mackay, I. R. Vulnerability of cell-surface receptors to autoimmune reactions. *Lancet,* 1975, 2 (7937), 684-687.

Carr, R. I., Shucard, D. W., Hoffman, S. A., Hoffman, A. W., Bardana, E. J., & Harbeck, R. J. Neuropsychiatric involvement in systemic lupus erythematosus. In D. Bergsma & A. L. Goldstein (Eds.), *International Symposium on Immunologic Components in Schizophrenia (1976: University of Texas Medical Branch at Galveston). Neurochemical and Immunologic Components in Schizophrenia.* (Birth defects. Original article series; vol. 14, no. 5). New York: Alan R. Liss, Inc., 1978, 209-235.

Cashman, N., Martin, C., Eizenbaum, J. F., Degos, J. D., & Bach, M. A. Monoclonal antibody-defining immunoregulatory cells in multiple sclerosis cerbrospinal fluid. *Journal of Clinical Investigation,* 1982, 70 (2), 387-392.

Charlesworth, J. A., Quin, J. W., & Yasmeen, D. Lymphocytotoxic antibodies in rheumatic diseases. In A. Maroudas & E. J. Holborow (Eds.), *Studies in Joint Disease II.* London: Pitman Medical, 1983, 57-87.

Crow, T. J. Positive and negative schizophrenic symptoms and the role of dopamine. *British Journal of Psychiatry,* 1981, 139, 251-254.

DeLisi, L. E., Weber, R. J., & Pert, C. B. Are there antibodies against brain in sera from schizophrenic patients? Review and prospectus. *Biological Psychiatry,* 1985, 20 (1), 110-115.

Dick, H. M., & Kissmeyer-Nielsen, F. (Eds.), *Histocompatibility Techniques.* Amsterdam: Elsevier, North Holland, 1979.

Dubois, E. L., Tallman, E., & Wonka, R. A. Chlorpromazine-induced systemic lupus erythematosus: Case report and review of the literature. *Journal of the American Medical Association,* 1972, 221 (6), 595-596.

Ellis, S. G., & Verity, M. A. Central nervous system involvement in systemic lupus erythematosus: A review of neuropathologic findings in 57 cases, 1955-1977. *Seminars in Arthritis and Rheumatism,* 1979, 8 (3), 212-221.

Farley, I. J., Price, K. S., McCullough, E., Deck, J. H., Hordynski, W., & Hornykeiwicz, O. Norepinephrine in chronic paranoid schizophrenia: Above-normal levels in limbic forebrain. *Science,* 1978, 200 (4340), 456-458.

Feinglass, E. J., Arnett, F. C., Dorsch, C. A., Zizic, T. M., & Stevens, M. B. Neuropsychiatric manifestations of systemic lupus erythematosus: Diagnosis, clinical spectrum, and relationship to other features of the disease. *Medicine (Baltimore),* 1976, 55 (4), 323-339.

Fessel, W. J. The "antibrain" factors in psychiatric patients' sera. I. Further studies with hemagglutination technique. *Archives of General Psychiatry,* 1963, 8 (6), 614-621.

Fessel, W. J. Autoimmunity and mental illness. A preliminary report. *Archives of General Psychiatry,* 1962, 6 (4), 320-323.

Fessel, W. J., Hirata-Hibi, M., & Shapiro, I. M. Genetic and stress factors affecting the abnormal lymphocyte in schizophrenia. *Journal of Psychiatric*

Research, 1965, 3 (4), 275-283.

Fieve, R. R., Blumenthal, B., & Little, B. The relationship of atypical lymphocytes, phenothiazines, and schizophrenia. *Archives of General Psychiatry,* 1966, 15 (5), 529-534.

Fontana, A., Fierz, W., & Wekerle, H. Astrocytes present myelin basic protein to encephalitogenic T-cell lines. *Nature (London),* 1984, 307 (5948), 273-276.

Fontana, A., Grieder, A., Arrenbrecht, S., & Grob, P. *In vitro* stimulation of glia cells by a lymphocyte-produced factor. *Journal of the Neurological Sciences,* 1980, 46 (1), 55-62.

Fudenberg, H. H., Whitten, H. D., Merler, E., & Farmati, O. Is schizophrenia an immunologic receptor disorder? *Medical Hypotheses,* 1983, 12 (1), 85-93.

Fujinami, R. S., & Oldstone, M. B. Amino acid homology between the encephalitogenic site of myelin basic protein and virus: Mechanism for autoimmunity. *Science,* 1985, 230 (4729), 1043-1045.

Fulford, K. W., Catterall, R. D., Delhanty, J. J., Doniach, D., & Kremer, M. A collagen disorder of the nervous system presenting as multiple sclerosis. *Brain,* 1972, 95 (2), 373-386.

Gershon, E. S., & Nurnberger, J. I. Inheritance of major psychiatric disorders. *Trends in Neurosciences,* 1982, 5 (7), 241-242.

Giulian, D., & Lachman, L. B. Interleukin-1 stimulation of astroglial proliferation after brain injury. *Science,* 1985, 228 (4698), 497-499.

Goldstein, A. L., Rossio, J., Kolyaskina, G. I., Emory, L. E., Overall, J. E., Thurman, G. B., & Hatcher, J. Immunological components in schizophrenia. In C. F. Baxter, & T. Melnechuk (Eds.), *Perspectives in Schizophrenia Research.* New York: Raven Press, 1980, 249-262.

Gottesman I. I., & Shields, J. *Schizophrenia and Genetics: A Twin Vantage Point.* New York: Academic Press, 1972.

Gottesman, I. I., & Shields, J. A critical review of recent adoption, twin, and family studies of schizophrenia: Behavioral genetics perspectives. *Schizophrenia Bulletin,* 1976, 2 (3), 360-401.

Gottlieb, P. M. Allergic neuropathies and demyelinative diseases. In F. Speer (Ed.), *Allergy of the Nervous System.* Springfield, Illinois: Charles C. Thomas, Publisher, 1970, 79-121.

Hafler, D. A., Fallis, R. J., Dawson, D. M., Schlossman, S. F., Reinherz, E. L., & Weiner, H. L. Immunologic responses of progressive multiple sclerosis patients treated with an anti-T-cell monoclonal antibody, anti-T12. *Neurology,* 1986, 36 (6), 777-784.

Hashim, G. A. Myelin basic protein: Structure, function and antigenic determinants. *Immunology Review,* 1978, 39, 60-107.

Hauser, S. L., Bahn, A. K., Gilles, F. H., Hoban, C. J., Reinherz, E. L.,

Schlossman, S. F., & Weiner, H. L. Immunohistochemical staining of human brain with monoclonal antibodies that identify lymphocytes, monocytes, and the Ia antigen. *Journal of Neuroimmunology,* 1983a, 5 (2), 197-205.

Hauser, S. L., Fosburg, M., Kevy, S., & Weiner, H. L. Plasmapheresis, lymphocytapheresis, and immunosuppressive drug therapy in multiple sclerosis. In R. S. A. Tindall (Ed.), *National Conference on Therapeutic Apheresis and Plasma Perfusion (3rd: 1982: Dallas, Texas). Therapeutic Apheresis and Plasma Perfusion.* New York: Alan T. Liss, 1982, 239-254.

Hauser, S. L., Reinherz, E. L., Hoban, C. J., Schlossman, S. F., & Weiner, H. L. Immunoregulatory T cells and lymphocytotoxic antibodies in active multiple sclerosis: Weekly analysis over a six-month period. *Annals of Neurology,* 1983b, 13 (4), 418-425.

Hauser, S. L., & Weiner, H. L. Cellular regulation of the human immune response and its relation to multiple sclerosis. In P. O. Behan & F. Spreafico (Eds.), *Neuroimmunology.* (Serono Symposia publications from Raven Press, Vol 12). New York: Raven Press, 1984, 247-259.

Heath, R. G., & Krupp, I. M. Schizophrenia as an immunologic disorder. I. Demonstration of antibrain globulins by fluorescent antibody techniques. *Archives of General Psychiatry,* 1967, 16 (1), 1-9.

Himmelhoch, J. M. What is schizophrenia? In D. Bergsma & A. L. Goldstein (Eds), *International Symposium on Immunologic Components in Schizophrenia (1976: University of Texas Medical Branch at Galveston). Neurochemical and Immunologic Components in Schizophrenia.* (Birth defects. Original article series; vol. 14, no. 5). New York: Alan R. Liss, Inc., 1978, 19-39.

Janković, B. D. Biological activity of antibrain antibody: An introduction to immunoneurology. In J. Gaito (Ed.), *Macromolecules and Behavior.* New York: Appleton-Century-Crofts, 1972, 99-130.

Janković, B. D. From immunoneurology to immunopsychiatry: Neuromodulating activity of anti-brain antibodies. *International Review of Neurobiology,* 1985a, 26, 249-314.

Janković, B. D. Neural tissue hypersensitivity in psychiatric disorders with immunologic features. *Journal of Immunology,* 1985b, 135 (2 Suppl.), 853s-857s.

Janković, B. D., Jakulić, S., & Horvat, J. Delayed skin hypersensitivity reactions to human brain S-100 protein in psychiatric patients. *Biological Psychiatry,* 1982, 17 (6), 687-697.

Janković, B. D., Jakulić, S., & Horvat, J. Schizophrenia and other psychiatric diseases: Evidence for neurotissue hypersensitivity. *Clinical and Experimental Immunology,* 1980, 40 (3), 515-522.

Janković, B. D., Rakić, L., Veskov, R., & Horvat, J. The effect of intraventricular injection of anti-brain antibody on defensive conditioned reflexes. *Nature (London)*, 1968, 218 (138), 270-271.

Jerne, N. K. Towards a network theory of the immune system. *Annales d' Immunologie (Paris)*, 1974, 125C (1-2), 373-389.

Jersild, C. The HLA system and multiple sclerosis. In D. Bergsma & A. L. Goldstein (Eds.), *International Symposium on Immunologic Components in Schizophrenia (1976: University of Texas Medical Branch at Galveston). Neurochemical and Immunologic Components in Schizophrenia.* (Birth defects. Original article series; vol. 14, no. 5). New York: Alan R. Liss, Inc., 1978, 123-170.

Johnson, K. P. Cerebrospinal fluid and blood assays of diagnostic usefulness in multiple sclerosis. *Neurology*, 1980, 30 (7, pt. 2), 106-109.

Kandel, E. R. Nerve cells and behavior. In E. R. Kandel & J. H. Schwartz (Eds.), *Principles of Neural Science.* 2nd Edition. New York: Elsevier/North-Holland, 1985, 13-24.

Khorshkho, V. K. *Reactii Zivotnogo Organizma na Vedenie Nervnoi Tkani (Nevrotoxini Anaphylaksia, Endotoxin).* Moscow, 1912.

Kinney, D. K., & Matthysse, S. Genetic transmission of schizophrenia. *Annual Review of Medicine*, 1978, 29, 459-473.

Kitamura, T. Dynamic aspects of glial reactions in altered brains. *Pathology, Research and Practice*, 1980, 168 (4), 301-343.

Knight, J. G. Dopamine receptor-stimulating autoantibodies: A possible cause of schizophrenia. *Lancet*, 1982, 2 (8307), 1073-1076.

Knight, J. G. Is schizophrenia an autoimmune disease? A review. *Methods and Findings in Experimental and Clinical Pharmacology*, 1984, 6 (7), 395-403.

Kolb, L. C. Relationship of demyelinating diseases to allergic encephalomyelitis. *Medicine (Baltimore)*, 1950, 29 (1), 99-121.

Kouzhetzova, N. F., & Seminov, S. F. Detection of antibrain antibodies in the blood serum of patients with neuropsychiatric diseases. *Zhurnal Nevropatologii i Psikhiatrii imeni S. S. Korsakov (Moskova)*, 1961, 61 (6), 869-874. (in Russian)

Lehmann-Facius, H. Serologisch-analytische Versuche mit Liquoren und Seren von Schizophrenien bezw. atypischen Psychosen. *Allgemeine Zeitschrift für Psychiatrie und Psychisch-Gerichtliche Medizin*, 1939, 110, 232-243.

Lindstrom, J. M., Seybold, M. E., Lennon, V. A., Whittingham, S., & Duane, D. D. Antibody to acetylcholine receptor in myasthenia gravis: Prevalence, clinical correlates, and diagnostic value. *Neurology*, 1976, 26 (11), 1054-1059.

Link, H., Möller, E., Muller, R., Norrby, E., Olsson, J. E., Stendahl, L., & Tibbling, G. Immunoglobulin abnormalities in spinal fluid in multiple sclerosis. *Acta Neurologica Scandinavica [Suppl.]*, 1977, 55 (63), 173-191.

Lisak, R. P. Antibodies to galactocerebroside: Probes for the study of antibody-determined neurologic damage. In P. O. Behan & F. Spreafico (Eds.), *Neuroimmunology.* (Serono Symposia publications for Raven Press, Vol. 12.) New York: Raven Press, 1984, 167-177.

Lisak, R. P., Zweiman, B., Burns, J. B., Rostami, A., & Silberberg, D. H. Immune responses to myelin antigens in multiple sclerosis. *Annals of the New York Academy of Sciences,* 1984, 436, 221-230.

McFarlin, D. E. Immunological abnormalities associated with neurological diseases. In P. O. Behan & F. Spreafico (Eds.), *Neuroimmunology.* (Serono Symposia publications for Raven Press, Vol. 12.) New York: Raven Press, 1984, 237-245.

McIntosh, R. M., Griswold, W. R., Koss, M. N. & Chernak, W. B. The choroid plexus: A possible role in autoimmune nephritis. *Clinical Research,* 1973, 21 (2), 324. (Abstract)

McIntosh, R. M., & Koss, M. M. The choroid plexus: Immunologic injury and disease. (Editorial) *Annals of Internal Medicine,* 1974, 81 (1), 111-113.

Meltzer, H. Y., & Stahl, S. M. The dopamine hypothesis of schizophrenia: A review. *Schizophrenia Bulletin,* 1976, 2 (1), 19-76.

Merrill, J. E., Myers, L. W., & Ellison, G. W. Cytotoxic cells in peripheral blood and cerebrospinal fluid of multiple sclerosis patients. *Annals of the New York Academy of Sciences,* 1984, 436, 192-205.

Mihailović, Lj., Divać, I., Mitrović, K., Milosević, D., & Janković, B. D. Effects of intraventricularly injected anti-brain antibodies on delayed alteration and visual discrimination tests performance in rhesus monkeys. *Experimental Neurology,* 1969, 24 (2), 325-336.

Mihailović, Lj., & Janković, B. D. Effects of intraventricularly injected anti-N. caudatus antibody on the electrical activity of the cat brain. *Nature (London),* 1961, 192 (4803), 665-666.

Möller, G. (Ed.), HLA and disease susceptibility. *Immunological Reviews,* 1983, 70. [Entire volume]

Morimoto, C., Reinherz, E. L., Schlossman, S. F., Schur, P. H., Mills, J. A., & Steinberg, A. D. Alterations in immunoregulatory T cell subsets in active systemic lupus erythematosus. *Journal of Clinical Investigation,* 1980, 66 (5), 1171-1174.

Norton, W. T. Formation, structure, and biochemistry of myelin. In G. J. Siegel, R. W. Albers, B. W. Agranoff, & R. Katzman (Eds.), *Basic Neurochemistry.* 3rd edition. Boston: Little, Brown and Co., 1981, 63-92.

Nurnberger, J. I., Jr., & Gershon, E. S. Genetics. In E. S. Paykel (Ed.), *Handbook of Affective Disorders.* New York: The Guilford Press, 1982, 126-145.

Nyland, H., Naess, A., & Lunde, H. Lymphocyte subpopulations in peripheral blood from schizophrenic patients. *Acta Psychiatrica Scandinavica (Den-*

mark), 1980, 61 (4), 313-318.

Patrick, J., & Lindstrom, J. Autoimmune response to acetylcholine receptor. *Science*, 1973, 180 (88), 871.

Prineas, J. W., & Wright, R. G. Macrophages, lymphocytes, and plasma cells in the perivascular compartment in chronic multiple sclerosis. *Laboratory Investigation*, 1978, 38 (4), 409-421.

Raveché, E. S. Genetics of human and murine lupus erythematosus. *NIH Conference. Systemic Lupus Erythematosus: Insights from Animal Models. Annals of Internal Medicine*, 1984, 100 (5), 714-716.

Reder, A. T., Antel, J. P., Oger, J. J., McFarland, T. A., Rosenkoetter, M., & Arnason, B. G. Low T_8 antigen density on lymphocytes in active multiple sclerosis. *Annals of Neurology*, 1984, 16 (2), 242-249.

Reich, W. The spectrum concept of schizophrenia. Problems for diagnostic practice. *Archives of General Psychiatry*, 1975, 32 (4), 489-498.

Richardson, E. P. Systemic lupus erythematosus. In P. J. Vinken & G. W. Bruyn (Eds.), *Handbook of Clinical Neurology: Neurological Manifestations of Systemic Disease*, Vol. 39, Part 2. Amsterdam: North Holland Publishing Co., 1980.

Rösler, M., Bellaire, W., Gressnich, N., Giannitsis, D., & Jarovici, A. HLA antigens in schizophrenia, major depressive disorder, and schizoaffective disorder. *Medical Microbiology and Immunology (Berlin)*, 1983, 172 (1) 57-65.

Russell, A. S. Drug induced autoimmune disease. In E. J. Holborow (Ed.), *Clinics in Immunology and Allergy*, Vol. 1, No. 1. London: W. B. Saunders Co., Ltd., 1981, 57-76.

Ryberg, B. Antibrain antibodies in multiple sclerosis: Relation to clinical variables. *Journal of Neurological Sciences*, 1982, 54 (2), 239-261.

Ryder, L. P., Platz, P., & Svejgaard, A. Histocompatibiity antigens and susceptibility to disease. Genetic considerations. In R. A. Reisfeld & S. Ferrone (Eds.), *Current Trends in Histocompatibility*, Vol. 2. New York: Plenum Press, 1981, 279-301.

Sandberg-Wollheim, M. Lymphocyte populations in the cerebrospinal fluid and peripheral blood of patients with multiple sclerosis and optic neuritis. *Scandanavian Journal of Immunology*, 1983, 17 (6), 575-581.

Schiffer, R. B., & Babigian, H. M. Behavioral disorders in multiple sclerosis, temporal lobe epilepsy, and amyotrophic lateral sclerosis. An epidemiologic study. *Archives of Neurology*, 1984, 41 (10), 1067-1069.

Schiffer, R. B., & Slater, J. R. Neuropsychiatric features of multiple sclerosis: Recognition and management. *Seminars in Neurology*, 5 (2), 1985, 127-133.

Schleifer, S. J., Keller, S. E., Siris, S. G., Davis, K. L., & Stein, M. Depression and immunity: Lymphocyte function in ambulatory depressed patients, hospitalized schizophrenic patients, and patients hospitalized for herniorrhaphy. *Archives of General Psychiatry,* 1985, 42 (2), 129-133.

Schwartz, R. H., Yano, A., & Paul, W. E. Interaction between antigen-presenting cells and primed T lymphocytes. An assessment of Ir gene expression in the antigen-presenting cell. *Immunology Reviews,* 1978, 40, 153-180.

Shapira, R., McKneally, S. S., Chou, F., & Kibler, R. F. Encephalitogenic fragment of myelin basic protein. Amino acid sequence of bovine, rabbit, guinea pig, monkey, and human fragments. *Journal of Biological Chemistry,* 1971, 246 (14), 4630-4640.

Solomon, G. F. Immunologic abnormalities in mental illness. In R. Ader (Ed.), *Psychoneuroimmunology.* New York: Academic Press, 1981, 259-278.

Spiegel, S., Fishman, P. H., & Weber, R. J. Direct evidence that endogenous GM1 ganglioside can mediate thymocyte proliferation. *Science,* 1985, 23 (4731), 1285-1287.

Speigel, S., Kassis, S., Wilchek, M., & Fishman, P. H. Direct visualization of redistribution and capping of fluorescent gangliosides on lymphocytes. *Journal of Cell Biology,* 1984, 99, (5), 1575-1581.

Stevens, J. R. The neuropathology of schizophrenia. (Editorial) *Psychological Medicine,* 1982, 12 (4), 695-700.

Swaak, A. J., Groenwold, J., Aarden, L. A., Statius van Eps, L. W., & Feltkamp, E. W. Prognostic value of anti-dsDNA in SLE. *Annals of the Rheumatic Diseases,* 1982, 41 (4), 388-395.

Tourtellotte, W. W., Potvin, A. R., Potvin, H. H., Ma, B. I., Baumhefner, R. W., & Syndulko, K. Multiple sclerosis *de novo* central nervous system IgG synthesis: Measurement, antibody profile, significance, eradication, and problems. In H. J. Bauer, S. Poser, & G. Ritter (Eds.), *Progress in Multiple Sclerosis Research.* New York: Springer-Verlag, 1980, 106-110.

Traugott, U., Reinherz, E. L., & Raine, C. S. Multiple sclerosis. Distribution of T cells, T cell subsets and Ia-positive macrophages in lesions of different ages. *Journal of Neuroimmunology,* 1983, 4 (3), 201-221.

Traugott, U., Stone, S. H., & Raine, C. S. Experimental allergic encephalomyelitis: Migration of early T cells from the circulation into the central nervous system. *Journal of Neurological Sciences.* 1978, 36, 55-61.

Trotter, J. L., & Brooks, B. R. Pathophysiology of cerebrospinal fluid immunoglobulins. In J. H. Wood (Ed.), *Neurobiology of Cerebrospinal Fluid.* New York: Plenum Press, 1980, 465-486.

Ullberg, M., & Jondal, M. Recycling and target binding capacity of human natural killer cells. *Journal of Experimental Medicine,* 1981, 153 (3), 615-628.

Waksman, B. H. Experimental allergic encephalomyelitis and the "auto-allergic" diseases. *International Archives of Allergy and Applied Immunology,* 1959, 14 [Suppl.], 1-87.

Walport, M. J., Fielder, A. H. , Batchelor, J. R., Black, C. M., Rynes, R. I., Dodi, I. T., & Hughes, G. R. HLA linked complement allotypes and genetic susceptibility to systemic lupus erythematosus (SLE). *Arthritis and Rheumatism,* 1982, 25 [Suppl.], 541. (Abstract)

Weiner, H. Schizophrenia: Etiology. In H. I. Kaplan & B. J. Sadock (Eds.), *Comprehensive Textbook of Psychiatry/IV.* 4th edition. Baltimore: Williams & Wilkins, 1985, 650-680.

Weiner, H. L., Bahn, A. K., Burks, J., Gilles, F., Kerr, C., Reinherz, E., & Hauser, S. L. Immunohistochemical analysis of the cellular infiltrate in multiple sclerosis lesions. *Neurology,* 1984a, 34 (3, Suppl. 1), 112.

Weiner, H. L., Hafler, D. A., Fallis, R. J., Johnson, D., Ault, K. A., & Hauser, S. L. T cell subsets in patients with multiple sclerosis. An overview. *Annals of the New York Academy of Sciences,* 1984b, 436, 281-293.

Weiner, H. L., & Hauser, S. L. Neuroimmunology I: Immunoregulation in neurological disease. *Annals of Neurology,* 1982, 11 (5), 437-449.

Wekerle, H., Linington, C., Lassmann, H., & Meyermann, R. Cellular immune reactivity within the CNS. *Trends in Neurosciences,* 1986, 9 (6), 271-277.

Whitaker, J. N. Antigenic determinants of myelin basic protein and its peptides. In P. O. Behan & F. Spreafico (Eds.), *Neuroimmunology.* (Serono Symposia publications from Raven Press, Vol. 12.) New York: Raven Press, 1984, 179-191.

Zarrabi, M. H., Zucker, S., Miller, F., Derman, R. M., Romano, G. S., Hartnett, J. A., & Varma, A. O. Immunologic and coagulation disorders in chlorpromazine-treated patients. *Annals of Internal Medicine,* 1979, 91 (2), 194-199.

BIBLIOGRAPHY

Bergsma, D., & Goldstein, A. L. (Eds.), *International Symposium on Immunologic Components in Schizophrenia (1976: University of Texas Medical Branch at Galveston). Neurochemical and immunologic components of schizophrenia.* (Birth defects. Original artical series; vol. 14, no. 5). New York: Alan R. Liss, Inc., 1978.

Carnegie, P. R., & Dunkley, P. R. Basic proteins of central and peripheral nervous system myelin. *Advances in Neurochemistry,* 1975, 1, 96-135.

Dick, H. M., & Kissmeyer-Nielsen, F. (Eds.), *Histocompatibility Techniques.* Amsterdam: Elsevier/North Holland, 1979.

Drachman, D. B. Myasthenia gravis. (First of two parts). *New England Journal of Medicine,* 1978, 298 (3), 136-142.

Drachman, D. B. Myasthenia gravis. (Second of two parts). *New England Journal of Medicine,* 1978, 298 (4), 186-193.

Gottesman, I. I., & Shields, J. A critical review of recent adoption, twin, and family studies of schizophrenia: Behavioral genetics perspectives. *Schizophrenia Bulletin,* 1976, 2 (3), 360-400.

Hashim, G. A. Myelin basic protein: Structure, function and antigenic determinants. *Immunology Review,* 1978, 39, 60-107.

Kandel, E. R., & Schwartz, J. H. *Principles of Neural Science.* 2nd edition. New York: Elsevier Scientific Publishing Co., Inc., 1985.

McFarlin, D. E., & McFarland, H. F. Multiple sclerosis. (First of 2 parts). *New England Journal of Medicine,* 1982, 307 (19), 1183-1188.

McFarlin, D. E., McFarland, H. F. Multiple sclerosis. (Second of 2 parts). *New England Journal of Medicine,* 1982, 307 (20), 1246-1251.

Meltzer, H. Y., & Stahl, S. M. The dopamine hypothesis of schizophrenia: A review. *Schizophrenia Bulletin,* 1976, 2 (1), 19-76.

Möller, G. (Ed.). HLA and disease susceptibility. *Immunological Reviews,* 1983, 70. [Entire volume]

Reich, W. The spectrum concept of schizophrenia. Problems for diagnostic practice. *Archives of General Psychiatry,* 1975, 32 (4), 489-498.

Wood, J. H. (Ed.) *Neurobiology of Cerebrospinal Fluid.* New York: Plenum Press, 1980.

Chapter 5

Experiential Effects on Immunity

> *Analyses of the interactions between behavior and the immune system are not a traditional part of either immunology or the behavioral or neurosciences, but perhaps they should be.*
>
> Robert Ader & Nicholas Cohen,
> *High Time for Psychoneuroimmunology,* 1985a.

In his earliest efforts to develop a concept that would explain the origin and course of what are now recognized as diseases of adaptation, Hans Selye was careful to note certain immunologic changes in his test animals (Selye, 1936, 1946). Hence, what he came to call the "general adaptation syndrome" included, as part of the syndrome, an involution of the thymus gland and lymph nodes, as well as downward shifts in both relative and absolute numbers of circulating leukocytes (Dalton & Selye, 1939; Harlow & Selye, 1937). Selye saw these changes as direct consequences of increased adrenal steroid outflow during the first stage (alarm reaction) of a three-stage physiologic response to acute physical stress.

It is unlikely that research design and execution in the "stress field" has become more rigorous and exacting with the passage of time. Yet, it is probably fair to say that scientists of the 80s confront a denser tangle of interacting variables than did their counterparts 50 years ago. It is of course a tangle of their own making, two reasons being obvious. To quote from Andrew A. Monjan's comprehensive resumé of research on stress and immunity in animals: "the last two decades have seen a phenomenal increase of knowledge concerning both brain-endocrine interactions and im-munology such that it would not be inappropriate to label earlier work as ancient history" (Monjan, 1981, p. 186). Then, too, today's investigators, unlike Selye, have introduced into their illustrative animal models be-havioral constructs that have greatly complicated their task. "Coping," "discrimination," "control," "dominance," "affiliation," and their opposite states, are typical of the intervening psychological variables that have be-come crucial to their schema.

Moreover, it is now established as incontrovertible that such subtle situational determinants as conflict, ambiguity, and uncertainty are of a kind to impose the ultimate "stress," especially when chronically ex-perienced. No less important are the repercussions on biological processes that can result from altering properties of one and the same psychologi-cally-relevant stimulus—its intensity, say, or duration.

NOTES ON MODEL-MAKING

Modern day stress research is carried out according to a number of procedural conventions that have developed gradually, by a process of slow accretion. Nowhere is this process more apparent than in the development of experimental model systems, components of which are routinely teased apart and reassembled in some newly optimum configura-tion, as might be done to an intricate mechanical device. The yoked ines-capable shock paradigm is one such experimental "apparatus." Exposure to moderate, randomly administered (hence unpredictable), inescapable (hence uncontrollable) electric shock is a predicament sufficiently daunt-ing to markedly alter an entire range of response in the affected organism. Its hormonal balance, the state of its emotions, its immunologic status, motor behavior, even its subsequent capacity to learn, are each influenced.

Psychoneuroimmunologists have taken it upon themselves to define complicated psychobiologic models of this general type at all levels, opt-ing for as wide-angled a perspective as possible, yet narrowing their scopes at will. They are thus challenged to occupy a theoretical space somewhere between abstract explanation, as exemplified, let us say, by general systems theory, and the empirical formats of scientific reduc-tionism (Cunningham, 1986). To grasp the mechanisms through which psychologic factors influence immunity is to take into account a series of energy transformations of stunning complexity within and between body systems. The encompassing view. By contrast, to study the psychoim-munopharmacology of the stress response, as that response is cir-cumscribed within the experimental shock paradigm, is to drastically constrict the visual field, adopting a rather telescopic line of reasoning in the process.

The inescapable shock paradigm has come into use as a basic laboratory tool in the study of motivated behavior, for despite its limitations, it has a number of dimensions relevant to some of the more general issues pertaining to stress and coping. For example, it is not enough to choose the type, duration, and severity of stressful stimulus most likely to elicit a particular psychophysiologic reaction pattern, without also taking into account the means, or lack of means, available to the animal subject to contend with a given stimulus condition. Likewise, it is not enough to record the waxing and waning of emotional response, without observing specific behaviors temporally associated with, and expressive of, that response. Learning effects embedded within the response complex (effects that may reflect the motive state and experiential history of the animal) must be extracted and analyzed, particularly under those circumstances (the more ideal) in which stress effects are monitored over time. The emotional and behavioral concomitants to conflict stress must then be juxtaposed against the stress-reactive dynamics of brain chemistry and the classic stress hormones (Mason, 1975a, 1975b), as well as against stress-related changes in the two reactive spheres of immunity, cellular and humoral (Cross et al., 1982; Riley, 1981; Shavit et al., 1984; Stein, Keller, & Schleifer, 1981).

In a general sense, the "coping" construct brings into relief the fundamental question of how crises of adaptation can affect health by undermining the psychic equanimity that is evidently basic to health (for discussions of this question, see Jemmott & Locke, 1984; Levy, 1984; Stein, Keller, Schleifer, 1985; Tecoma & Huey, 1985). In a more restricted sense, the construct is used in this chapter as an expedient device with which to recapitulate our thesis. For it will become evident that each of the physiologic response systems with which we have been concerned throughout the text are affected in some way by the adaptive stratagems of coping.

That is not to say that all consequences of the coping paradigm make for a smooth fit. Learning (i.e., conditioning) effects and the analgesic reaction are two likely consequences of the "noncoping" predicament that have been studied as separate phenomena from the separate orientations of behavioral psychology and opioid peptide research. Yet, whereas each of these two areas of study has at last made connection to the field of immunology, neither has made connection to the other.

These weak links notwithstanding, the coping model illustrates dramatically the interplay between emotion and immunity in adaptation. It is obvious that, to have successfully adapted, an organism must have attained its own particular compromise between accommodation and initiative. It must, in a manner of speaking, have struck a balance between reactive orientation to change and purposeful action as agent to change. By means of the coping model, this chapter sets forth a rationale for psycho-neuroimmunology from observations of immune competency in humans and animals that are thwarted in either one or both of these two complementary tendencies.

Learning is intrinsic to adaptation. Our defense of this rationale begins, therefore, with a brief discussion of *immunologic* adaptation. We will present but a small part of the evidence showing that discriminative responses of the immune system, like all other adaptive physiological responses of the organism, operate in accordance with the basic principles of learning (for full review articles on the behavioral conditioning of the immune response, see Ader, 1985b; Ader & Cohen, 1981, 1985b).

We shall then discuss several of the model systems from animal research that have strongly impacted on the development of psycho-neuroimmunology. Towards the close of this discussion, we shall be returning to the subject of the opioid peptides, this time from a different perspective. We shall not only be illustrating the singular sensitivity of opioid systems to the psychologic dimensions of specific stressors, but will also attempt to portray the range of psychoneuroimmunologic response affected by these systems under conditions of stress.

Finally, and inevitably, we must address the question of relevance. How relevant are animal models and the constraints of laboratory "environments" to human experience?

CONDITIONING AND THE IMMUNE RESPONSE

Behavioral research is rooted in the premise that learning is a form of adaptation, and—as corollary to this premise—that classical and instrumental conditioning are forms of learning. Were these postulates to be restated in the schematic of actual experiment, one would say that a random stimulus, once innocuous in its neutrality, takes on significance only to the extent to which its occurrence is contiguous both with the organisms's response to its occurrence, and with the consequences of that response, overt or otherwise. The accuracy and strength of this association are then understood to predetermine the organism's future ability to predict, to resolve conflict, even to make the instrumental choices that will assure its well-being and survival—in a word, to adapt.

Understood in this context, the expression of emotion can be considered a specific conditioned response, entrained to a generalized, innate, species-specific stress response. From what we know of the interactions of systems, we can deduce that the immune response is but one, among several, interoceptive response systems operating within this response complex. Indeed, when the response capacity of the immune system is viewed in this way, as a part of the totality of adaptive response, it seems extraordinary that proof of immune conditionability should have been so long a matter of controversy (Ader, 1981; Luk'ianenko, 1961).

It will be recalled that research on the behavioral conditioning of immunity has had a long and uneven history, beginning with first studies of behavioral immunology at l'Institut Pasteur in Paris in the 1920s (Ader, 1981). The many differences in experimental approach in studies undertaken since that time—differences in choice of situational variables, choice of stimuli, schedules of contingency, choice of variables particular to the host, etc.—have only helped to confirm that learned immunologic response is both replicable and generalizable (Ader & Cohen, 1981, 1985b).

Unconditioned stimuli have included the administration of toxins, ionizing radiation, and the injection of antigen. Conditioned stimuli, both appetitive and aversive, have included novel taste, noise stress, and electric shock. Conditioned immunologic response has been measured by such immune parameters as graft-versus-host (GvH) reaction to allogeneic skin graft, T and B cell response to mitogen, humoral antibody response, mast cell histamine release, natural killer (NK) cell reactivity, and lymph node weight.

A typical instance of single trial learning, observed in a routine conditioning experiment carried out in an American laboratory in the 1970s, at once provided the historic link to the earlier work of the Russians, the prototype to later work, and the impetus to renewed interest in the psychologic dimension of the immune response. Robert Ader and Nicholas Cohen (1975) set up a prototype experiment after having made the "serendipitous observation" that mortality increased in rats during conditioning trials that were programmed to extinguish an acquired taste aversion to a substance first associated with an illness-inducing, immunosuppressive drug.

According to the prototype, conditioned immunosuppression is initially established by the single pairing of an innocuous gustatory stimulus with illness-induced taste aversion. Specifically, presentation of sodium saccharin, acting as conditioned stimulus (CS), is temporally associated with the intraperitoneal injection of the aversive drug, cyclophosphamide, acting as unconditioned stimulus (US). The acquisition of conditioned immunosuppression is then evident in a depressed hemagglutinin antibody titer serving as the measure of conditioned response (CR) to antigen (i.p. injection of sheep red blood cells [SRBC]) presented in association with the once-innocuous, now behaviorally significant, conditioned stimulus (saccharin).

One obvious reason for the revival of interest in this specialized area of immunology is the potential clinical relevance of the findings (Ader, 1985a, 1985b). It has been shown, for instance, how an immunosuppressive conditioning protocol, as tested in an animal model of systemic lypus erythematosus (the female New Zealand [NZBxNZW]F$_1$ mouse), might be introduced to advantage in the treatment of this autoimmune (hyperimmune) disorder in humans (Ader & Cohen, 1982).

The direct conditioned *enhancement* of host resistance has also been demonstrated. The temporal pairing of exposure to an odor (camphor) with injection of a therapeutic drug (poly-inosine:poly-cytidylic acid [poly I:C]) has been shown to increase NK cell activity in inbred female Balb/c mice, as evidenced by percent chromium[51] release (Ghanta et al., 1985).

VARIATIONS ON A THEME: THE "COPING PARADIGM"

Research to date has shown that loss of initiative in the face of challenge, or, alternatively, loss of the capacity to accommodate to challenge—essentially the loss of control, or *perceived* loss of control over external events—constitute sources of stress. Controllability and predictability are in fact stimulus dimensions of such potency that under experimental conditions in which either one or both are absent (or lost, once attained), an animal subject is likely to be rendered helpless (for comprehensive review, see Mineka & Henderson, 1985).

Researchers find that when stimulus occurrence and the animal's response to the stimulus are so programmed as to be independent of one another, the animal quickly learns that its best efforts in its own defense are irrelevant, that it is without resource (Overmier & Wielkiewicz, 1983). They find also that, having lost dominion over events that are vital to its self-interest, the animal is likely to manifest the certain signs and symptoms of adaptive failure under new and different circumstances of threat. In a word, it has *learned* to be helpless (Maier & Seligman, 1976; Overmier & Seligman, 1967; Seligman et al., 1980).

Certain kinds of social forces can act as especially acute stressors. Of these, some few are now reproducible and manipulable in the laboratory. Social forces tend to be universal. Consequently, findings on the psychobiology of animals so stressed are seen as broadly applicable to the human condition—the phylogenetic gulf separating the species notwithstanding.

Even so benign an example of psychosocial stress as displacement within the hierarchy of a nonhuman primate group becomes, when recast in human terms, the disrupted exercise of personal control, frustration in the realization of self-efficacy (Bandura, 1985) or, as seen in human male subjects, inhibition of the power motive (McClelland et al., 1980). To the psychoneuroimmunologist, parallels of particular interest reside in the fact that similar neurohormonal and immunologic patterns of response mirror similar kinds of stressful experience in different species. Loss of "status" in the animal heirarchy or, alternatively, the diminished sense of self-efficacy—hence, diminished social preeminence—in humans, are kindred stressors that have served to illustrate such parallels.

More than this, new data are now indicating that acute psychologic states marked by powerlessness, conflict, or threat can place organisms at risk in a special sense; which is to say that reactive elements within the immune system reflect, with remarkable fidelity, the success or failure of adaptive strategies of control.

Psychologic vulnerability appears to be linked to neurochemical imbalance and to salient behavioral attitudes and postures, as well as to adverse changes in immune status. The study of these correlations has become a research priority, one that is made easier by conspicuous analogies between human and animal reactions to psychologic and psychosocial stress.

Analogy in Stress Research

In a 1980 study, Geraldine Cassens and her colleagues found that a single exposure to moderately intense inescapable footshock, administered on a variable interval schedule, produced a significant increase in the level of norepinephrine (NE) metabolite (MHPH-SO$_4$) in the brain of the rat. A like increase occurred following reexposure of the animal solely to the environmental stimulus context associated with this one isolated experience of shock. The neurometabolic shift was accompanied, in each instance, by such behavioral indices of emotion as crouching and postural rigidity.

In a similar study, again employing an uncontrollable stressor and the laboratory rat as animal subject, Jay M. Weiss and coworkers (1981) found NE stores to be depleted in the locus coeruleus region of the brain, and noted, as well, a "behavioral depression" in the shocked animals. In still another study that has used a virtually identical shock/stress paradigm, again tested in the rat, MacLennan and Maier (1983) found amphetamine sulfate and cocaine-induced behavioral stereotypy to occur only in those animals unable to control the delivery of shock, both groups, experimental and control, having received identical shocks and identical doses of drug.

In the Cassens study, the elevation in brain metabolite and the animal's stereotyped behavioral response were seen, in combination, as a non-specific anticipatory defense reaction to a specific stimulus *milieu*, which, as conditional stimulus, assumed a predictive value, arousing the expectation of shock. Each of these studies, however, illustrates the survival value of emotion. It may be presumed, that is to say, that in each of the three, reexposure to the ambience of experienced peril would most probably reelicit the original emotion in some of its original intensity, recalled emotion then serving as cue to alert the animal to its own vulnerability in a circumstance beyond its control.

Given the psychologic vulnerability which it appears capable of engendering in animals, the paradigm of learned helplessness has been under careful study as a model for clinical depression in humans (Porsolt et al., 1978; Seligman, 1974, 1975; Sherman et al., 1979). In a restricted sense, the model fits. In regard to neurochemical mediation alone, for example, an approximate analogy can be found in the neuroendocrine imbalance that has long been known to be symptomatic of endogenous depression in humans (Sachar, 1975). Furthermore, although it may not adequately reflect the heterogeneity of the clinical syndrome, the model suggests the degree to which failure to cope can operate as a precipitating factor in certain subtypes of depressive illness (Maier, 1984).

Indeed, when so utilized, the fitness of the model is striking. By way of illustration, rats, pretreated with an anxiety-producing benzodiazepine receptor ligand (β-carboline, N-methyl-β-carboline-3-carboxamide [FG-7142]), are blocked in the acquisition of avoidance behavior following inescapable tailshock. On the other hand, learned helplessness does not develop in those animals pretreated with a tranquilizing drug ($[^3H]$Ro 15 1788) that acts as a selective antagonist to central benzodiazepine binding sites (Drugan et al., 1985).

Separation stress in primates is another experimental animal model that is applicable to human beings. An initial agitation, followed by depression and seeming helplessness, is a characteristic behavioral sequence in infant monkeys during maternal separation (Coe et al., 1984; Kalin & Carnes, 1984; Reite, 1977; Suomi, Collins, & Harlow, 1973; Suomi, Mineka, & LeLizio, 1983). The identical behavioral sequence has been noted in human infants undergoing comparable separation anxiety (Field & Reite, 1984).

Most important, given our underlying theme, is the finding that "depressed" infant monkeys, separated from their mothers or peers, show reductions in immune competence (Coe et al., 1984; Laudenslager, Reite, & Harbeck, 1982; Reite, Harbeck, & Hoffman, 1981). Of comparable interest is the recent report by Mark Laudenslager and his group that compromised immunity persists into the adulthood of monkeys subjected to temporary maternal and peer separation in infancy (Laudenslager, Capitanio, & Reite, 1985). This latter finding is the more interesting in the light of earlier evidence (Solomon, 1968) that rat pups, exposed daily for 21 days post-parturition to brief (3 minute) handling and novel environment, showed significantly greater elevation in primary and secondary antibody response to antigen (flagellin polymer) in adulthood than did unhandled animals.

Interesting findings indeed, but it is obvious that at least three different stressors are subject to confounding in studies of this kind: one, the stress of handling; two, the stress of separation; three, the stress of exposure to unfamiliar surroundings. Moreover, either the duration, and/or periodicity, of any one of these stressors, in interaction with subject variables, could alone explain the opposite immunologic effects obtained.

Experiential effects on immunity find a likely parallel in human infants in the deteriorative outcome of maternal separation and abandonment known as "failure to thrive" (Cupoli, Hallock, & Barness, 1980). It is to be assumed (though not yet proven) that this critical psychophysiologic condition is marked by a generalized dysfunction of the immune system.

Conjugal bereavement is a kindred stressor experienced in human adulthood that is typically characterized both by reactive depression and immune suppression (Bartrop et al., 1977; Schleifer et al., 1983). This discovery is congruent with evidence that patients with major depressive illness show signs of immune impairment, i.e., lymphopenia and diminished lymphocyte stimulation response, as assessed *in vitro* (Kronfol et al., 1985; Schleifer et al., 1984, 1985).

It can be argued that separation stress in the very young, of whatever species, is a radical abrogation of the coping response. Deprived of maternal support and comfort, but most importantly, the primary contingent relationship of infancy, the infant is likewise deprived of its one and only agent of control over its world, however indirect and fragile the exercise of that control (Ainsworth, 1982; Levine, 1980). It can also be argued that the pain of bereavement must reflect, in considerable degree, the loss of a crucial "contingent relationship" in adult life.

Other state-dependent measures, not unrelated to separation stress, have a comparably negative influence on immune function, indicating that compromised immunity and various forms of alienation are somehow intertwined. As a case in point, a relative lack of affiliation with others, the inner need for power over others, combined with the frustration of that power, are associated both with an increased incidence of illness (McClelland & Jemmott, 1980; McClelland et al., 1980) and diminished immune competence, as indicated by low levels of secretory immunoglobulin A (S-IgA) (Jemmott et al., 1983; McClelland, Alexander, & Marks, 1982).

A concordant finding is reported by Janice K. Kiecolt-Glaser and colleagues, who have shown that loneliness in young adults, as evaluated in self-report (UCLA Loneliness Scale), is inversely correlated with immune efficacy (in this case, a diminution in natural killer cell activity) (Kiecolt-Glaser et al., 1984a, 1984b).

The telling factor in psychosocial studies of this kind is the degree to which emotional and perceptual overlay alters the objective reality of stressful life events (Locke & Kraus, 1982; Locke et al., 1984). Animal research offers some striking illustrations of this phenomenon. For instance, the "social buffering" of conspecifics in primate groups has a direct effect on plasma cortisol secretion during exposure of the animals to a conditioned fear stimulus, the intensity of the stimulus remaining constant. Stanton, Patterson, and Levine (1985) have shown steroid output in monkeys to increase in direct correspondence to increased social isolation, the least output in the group condition, a greater output in the dyad condition, greatest output in the solitary condition. A similar phenomenon has been reported in mice, where performance deficits following inescapable shock were found to be far more pronounced in isolated, than in grouped, mice (Anisman & Sklar, 1981).

OPIOID PEPTIDES IN REACTION CHAINS

Social defeat in rodents is yet another laboratory model that demonstrates dramatically the biological complexity of failed coping and the vulnerable state. When repeatedly subjected to physical attack from a mouse of another strain, the laboratory mouse will neither retaliate against, nor escape, its tormentor. Instead, the afflicted animal adopts a species-specific posture of submission, a posture that is characterized by rigidity, immobility, and analgesia (Miczek & O'Donnell, 1978; Miczek, DeBold, & Thompson, 1984; Miczek, Thompson, & Shuster, 1982). Another study of psychogenic analgesia, again produced in mice, again accompanied by submission and "appeasement gestures," shows the increased serum corticosterone levels that would be expected to occur as part of a generalized stress response (Leshner, Merkel, & Mixon, 1982).

This latter report notwithstanding, the consensus view is that analgesia is centrally (i.e., neurally) mediated by endogenous opiate peptide transmitters acting through pain-inhibitory circuits in the brain and spinal cord. Neither hypophysectomy, adrenalectomy, nor total sympathetic blockade attenuates the analgesic response (Watkins et al., 1982). Additionally, defeat-induced analgesia in adrenalectomized mice is blocked by microinjection of an opiate antagonist (naloxone) into the arcuate nucleus of the hypothalamus and the periaqueductal grey area of the brain (Miczek, Thompson, & Shuster, 1985).

We will not digress to describe these very complex opioid-mediated pain-inhibitory systems other than to point out the following facts as background to the points we wish to raise with regard to these systems and behavior:

1. Two classes of opioid peptides, the endorphins and enkephalins, cleaved from three related precursor peptide molecules, proopiomelanocortin (POMC), proenkephalin, and prodynorphin, make up three widely distributed networks in the central nervous system (Dupont et al., 1980; Fitzgerald, 1986; Fraioli, Isidori, & Mazzetti, 1984; Khachaturian et al., 1985).

2. In association with these networks are multiple stereoselective opioid receptors or recognition sites, which mediate differing effects, depending upon their tissue locus and chemical configuration (Watkins, Cobelli, & Mayer, 1982).

3. Opiate and nonopiate receptors are both involved in pain perception (nociception) (Gebhart, 1982; Watkins & Mayer, 1982). The two receptor subtypes are distinguishable on the basis of their reaction to morphine, this exogenous opiate being an agonist of the opiate receptor, but not of the nonopiate receptor.

4. Additionally, opiate antagonists, such as naloxone and naltrexone, selectively block the opiate receptor, but have no affect upon the nonopiate receptor.

5. Molecular structure can be a determinant of these differential effects. In the β-endorphin molecule, for example, the N-terminal fragment is locus to opioid receptor recognition or binding, and is naloxone-sensitive; the carboxy terminus, on the other hand, is locus to nonopiate-mediated receptor binding and is insensitive to naloxone.

6. Putting it another way, morphine acts as a "marker" for the opioid, narcotic form of stress-induced analgesia, but not for a second, equally potent, nonnaloxone-sensitive, nonnarcotic form of analgesia mediated by nonopioid receptor components (for a detailed reviews of opioid receptor structure and chemical affinity, see Chang, 1984; Moretti et al., 1984).

7. To add complication to an already complicated picture, differential shock effects can be a function of *body* locus: the analgesic reaction in the rat, for example, will differ depending upon the area stimulated, whether front paw, hind paw, or all four paws (for review of these data, see Watkins et al., 1982; Watkins, Cobelli, & Mayer, 1982).

The analgesic reaction to noxious stimulation is psychologically, as well as physiologically, complex. As we have seen in the case of conditioned norepinephrine release (Cassens et al., 1980), stimulus generalization effects (i.e., contextual cues associated with an initial experience of shock) can evoke analgesia in a previously shocked animal (Sherman et al., 1984; Watkins, Cobelli, & Mayer, 1982). What is more, an exquisite margin of discrimination exists between the two forms of analgesia, opioid *versus* nonopioid, with respect to the behavioral outcome of aversive stimulation. For instance, opiate-mediated analgesia occurs in rats unable to escape (control) electric footshock, but not in those animals responding to the escapable shock condition (see Maier, 1984, for general review).

An equally intriguing finding is that stimulus parameters, such as shock duration and intensity, operate as sensitive criteria for the selective activation of opioid pathways. For example, prolonged, intermittent footshock produces the opioid-mediated form of analgesia, whereas exposure to brief, continuous footshock produces the nonopioid form of analgesia (Maier, 1984). The idea that learning (under the prolonged stimulus condition) might be producing the differential effect (Maier, 1984) has been thought questionable, in view of the fact that opiate analgesia also occurs in decerebrate animals exposed to prolonged shock (Watkins et al., 1984).

Of the two forms of analgesia, only the opioid-mediated form elicited in reaction to inescapable electric shock has proven to be immunosuppressive, as evidenced by decreased natural killer (NK) cell cytotoxicity (Shavit et al., 1984) and enhanced tumor development (Shavit et al., 1983; Visintainer, Volpicelli, & Seligman, 1982). Comparable to its effect upon pain-inhibitory pathways, the opioid effect upon immunity is centrally mediated. Accordingly, the direct injection of morphine into the right lateral ventricle of the brain suppresses NK cytotoxicity, an effect that is blocked by the opiate receptor antagonist, naltrexone. By contrast, the systemic administration of N-methylmorphine, a morphine analogue that does not cross the blood-brain barrier, has no influence on NK activity (Shavit et al., 1986).

Notable in this context is the discovery that opioids inhibit the production of interferon, a lymphokine that is stimulatory to NK cells (Silva, Bonavida, & Targan, 1980). As might be expected, morphine has also been found to block interferon production (Hung, Lefkowitz, & Geber, 1973).

In summary, these many threads of evidence can be gathered together to compose a total picture. One: the state of opioid stress analgesia, triggered in reaction to intermittent, inescapable shock, is an immunologically compromised condition. Two: this form of analgesia, and the particular immune dysfunction with which it is associated, are brought about through the activation of opioid peptide pathways within the central nervous system. Three: opioid-mediated analgesia is associated with learned help-lessness and may, by consequence, also be defined as a psychologically compromised condition (for detailed reviews of this literature, see Maier et al., 1983; Minor, Jackson, & Maier, 1984; Shavit et al., 1985; Terman et al., 1984).

MODELS WITHIN LIMITS

Investigators hope, of course, that in the coping paradigm and the com-posite stress profile that "inescapability" typically evokes, they will have directly targeted some of the psychophysiologic antecedents of disease. They may in fact be close to their goal. For one thing, they have been as-sisted in their quest by a working model that affords a generous latitude for inference. For another, by operating from a structured frame of reference, they have been emboldened to ask how conditions of stress, en-countered "in the field," might be reducible to critical components of the model.

There can hardly be a better argument in favor of the utility of models than the foregoing demonstration of covariance between environmental conditions and their physiologic and psychologic consequences. We have seen a single stimulus attribute, such as uncontrollability, bring about pronounced changes in brain activity, steroid hormone output, immune ac-tivity, and emotional status, as well as influence concurrent and on-going behavior.

Yet, ironically, the very ingenuity of these laboratory facsimiles of human experience has been instrumental in better defining "the human fac-tor," in emphasizing the full implication of phylogeny. By their having been brought so expertly into relief by model systems, similarities of response between species have helped to articulate crucial areas of differ-ence. It is in the nature of these differences that researchers believe they may have isolated uniquely human attributes that exert an especial in-fluence on stress tolerance and health behavior.

Although there has been relatively little research along these lines, some interesting theories are beginning to take shape. In a series of empirical studies that are a model of painstaking theory-building, Martin E.P. Seligman and coworkers have taken as subjects for analysis: first, the manner in which stressful life events are subjectively evaluated by dif-ferent individuals; and second, the ways in which interpretive sets of this kind can impact upon future well-being. Their data have shown how pain-ful emotional experience is cognitively, idiosyncratically, reformulated by the psyche; how, as a set of explanatory, intrinsically logical constructs, this reformulation can then affect future behavior in the face of similarly, and even dissimilarly, painful experience (Alloy et al., 1984). In the depressed individual, for example, this reformulation or "explanatory style" typically takes on a fatalistic caste reinforcing to the sense of helplessness, diminished self-esteem, and the tendency to self-blame so characteristic of the condition (Peterson & Seligman, 1984).

There are investigators who have analyzed cognitive styles of coping from a more positive perspective. Objecting to the limitations of the helplessness model, Rothbaum, Weisz, and Snyder (1982) have argued that individuals go to great lengths to devise strategies of accomodation, marshalling "a broad range of inward behaviors" with which to overcome the perceived loss of control, and the sense of powerlessness associated with that perception.

Shelley E. Taylor has countered the helplessness model with the thesis that human powers of adjustment to life's adversities are remarkable in their persistence and flexibility, particularly with respect to the advantageous uses of illusion: the "effective individual in the face of threat, then, seems to be one who permits the development of illusions, nurtures those illusions, and is ultimately restored by those illusions" (Taylor, 1983, p. 1168).

Suzanne C. Kobasa's concept of "hardiness" (Kobasa, 1979; Kobasa, Makki, & Kahn, 1982), and the salutary consequences to health ("salutogenesis") of what Anton Antonovsky (1981, 1984) has called a "sense of coherence," are other contributions to the general thesis that, depending upon its nature, an individual's subjective orientation to the external world can provide a protective buffer against the stresses of life. It is refreshing, in this regard, to come upon Neal E. Miller's reminder that "laughter, beauty, love, affection" are transcendent elements of vitality and health, but disquieting, too, to realize that the mechanisms of their influence remain largely unexplored (Miller, 1983).

Even so, the potential powers for healing in mind, spirit, and the imagination are slowly becoming the province of medical science. Interest grows in the therapeutic uses of hypnosis in psychiatry (Bowers & Kelly, 1979) and clinical medicine (Barber, 1978; Wadden & Anderson, 1982). The beneficial effects of directed imagery (autohypnosis) are also gaining the attention of the medical community (Holden, 1978; Olness, 1981; Simonton, Matthews-Simonton, & Creighton, 1978; Simonton, Matthews-Simonton, & Sparks, 1980).

As might be expected, there is "scientific" skepticism towards data that, to date, have been largely anecdotal. Indirect, objective measures of hormonal and immunologic change correlative to evoked psychological states (Rogers, Dubey, & Reich, 1979; Sachar, Cobb, & Shor, 1966) will no doubt temper that skepticism, in time, and to some degree (see Hall, 1982-1983, for recent review). A most radical shift in emphasis in medical research will be required, however, if effects upon health of an individual's subjective orientation to the *internal* world are to be acknowledged as "legitimate and real" (Epstein, 1986).

CONCLUSIONS

To say that the immune system is a partner in adaptation is to state the obvious. What has been less than obvious until now is the immediacy of immune involvement in adaptation. A purpose of this final review chapter has been to describe some of the psychosocial conditions, both in and out of the laboratory, that emphasize this aspect of immunity.

A second purpose has been to consider how emotions, percepts, and cognitions, the stuff of primary experience, become reflected in the purely *physiologic* domain; more than that, how distortion and bias within the one, purely psychologic, domain can either favorably, or adversely, affect outcomes in body systems. Models of adaptation in animals devised for the study of adaptation in humans, though limited in critical ways, bring certain particulars into relief that bear on this puzzling question. They do this by revealing relationships. In addition, they emphasize the *pattern* of relationships between systems in organisms experiencing distress.

Perhaps most importantly, biopsychosocial models are a showcase for the effects of learning. There is no reason not to suppose that each of the variables involved in psychogenic stress is subject to conditioning, the few examples cited in this review by no means exhausting the list.

Learning operates in both domains, physiologic and psychologic. Learning implies more or less permanent change in infrastructures supporting both domains. Learning also implies changes in habit: habits of physiologic response, habits of thought, *habits of immunologic response*, some adaptive, some less so.

The question that begs asking, at this juncture, is whether there is not an operant within the immune repertoire. Is there not a means whereby the response systems of immunity could be conditioned *instrumentally*? All physiological processes are, by nature, spontaneously variable, immune processes being no exception in this regard. Given this characteristic, it is conceivable that a "right" immune response could become the operant to reinforcement, to reward.

One might ask, in other words, if there is not an immune process sensitive to psychological manipulation and control through external feedback, as has been demonstrated in the operant control of other bodily processes.

Or, to turn the question around, could selective changes in other physio-logical response systems produced through feedback influence the immune system?

Here, serendipity might again enter the picture. There is that chance that by manipulating one palpably manipulable response, physiologic or psy-chologic, investigators may gain indirect access to a single response com-ponent of the immune system, finding in the two an exact covariance.

The immune system produces psychoactive peptides. What input might these hormones have on the conditioning of the system itself? And to what extent do "signal molecules" of the immune system contribute to the con-ditioning of other systems?

These questions follow as a matter of course from the material reviewed in this book. That they can be asked at all is a testament to the rapidity with which discoveries in psychoneuroimmunology are becoming in-tegrated into other orbits of biological science.

REFERENCES

Ader, R. An historical account of conditioned immunologic responses. In R. Ader (Ed.), *Psychoneuroimmunology.* New York: Academic Press, 1981, 321-352.

Ader, R. Conditioned immunopharmacologic effects in animals: Implications for a conditioning model of pharmacotherapy. In L. White, B. Tursky, & G. E. Schwartz (Eds.), *Placebo: Theory, Research, and Mechanisms.* New York: The Guilford Press, 1985a, 306-323.

Ader, R. Conditioned taste aversions and immunopharmacology. *Annals of the New York Academy of Sciences,* 1985b, 443, 293-307.

Ader, R., & Cohen, N. Behaviorally conditioned immunosuppression. *Psychosomatic Medicine,* 1975, 37 (4), 333-340.

Ader, R., & Cohen, N. Conditioned immunopharmacological responses. In R. Ader (Ed.), *Psychoneuroimmunology.* New York: Academic Press, 1981, 281-319.

Ader, R., & Cohen, N. Behaviorally conditioned immunosuppression and murine systemic lupus erythematosus. *Science,* 1982, 215 (4539), 1534-1536.

Ader, R., & Cohen, N. High time for psychoneuroimmunology. *Nature (London),* 1985a, 315 (6015), 103-104.

Ader, R., & Cohen, N. CNS-immune system interactions: Conditioning phenomena. *Behavior and Brain Sciences,* 1985b, 8 (3), 379-395.

Ainsworth, M. D. Attachment: Retrospect and prospect. In C. M. Parkes & J. Stevenson-Hinde (Eds.), *The Place of Attachment in Human Behavior.* New

York: Tavistock Publications, 1982, 3-30.

Alloy, L. B., Peterson, C., Abramson, L. Y., & Seligman, M. E. P. Attributional style and the generality of learned helplessness. *Journal of Personality and Social Psychology,* 1984, 46 (3), 681-687.

Anisman, H., & Sklar, L. S. Social housing conditions influence escape deficits produced by uncontrollable stress: Assessment of the contribution of norepinephrine. *Behavioral and Neural Biology,* 1981, 32 (4), 406-427.

Antonovsky, A. *Health, Stress, and Coping.* San Francisco: Jossey-Bass Publishers, 1979.

Antonovsky, A. The sense of coherence as a determinant of health. *Advances,* 1984, 1 (3), 37-50.

Bandura, A., Taylor, C. B., Williams, S. L., Mefford, I. N., & Barchas, J. D. Catecholamine secretion as a function of perceived coping self-efficacy. *Journal of Consulting and Clinical Psychology,* 1985, 53 (3), 406-414.

Barber, T. X. Hypnosis, suggestions and psychosomatic phenomena: A new look from the standpoint of recent experimental studies. *American Journal of Clinical Hypnosis,* 1978, 21 (1), 13-25.

Bartrop, R. W., Luckhurst, E., Lazarus, L., & Kiloh, L. G., & Penny, R. Depressed lymphocyte function after bereavement. *Lancet,* 1977, 1 (8016), 834-836.

Bowers, K. S., & Kelly, P. Stress, disease, psychotherapy and hypnosis. *Journal of Abnormal Psychology,* 1979, 88 (5), 490-505.

Cassens, G., Roffman, M., Kuruc, A., Orsulak, P. J., & Schildkraut, J. J. Alterations in brain norepinephrine metabolism induced by environmental stimuli previously paired with inescapable shock. *Science,* 1980, 209 (4461), 1138-1140.

Chang, K. J. Opioid receptors: Multiplicity and sequelae of ligand-receptor interactions. In P. M. Conn (Ed.), *The Receptors,* Vol. I. Orlando: Academic Press, 1-81.

Coe, C. L., Wiener, S. G., Rosenberg, L. T., & Levine, S. Endocrine and immune responses to separation and maternal loss in non-human primates. In M. Reite & T. Fields (Eds.), *The Psychobiology of Attachment.* New York: Academic Press, 1984, 163-199.

Cross, R. J., Brooks, W. H., Roszman, T. L., & Markesbery, W. R. Hypothalamic-immune interactions. Effect of hypophysectomy on neuroimmunomodulation. *Journal of Neurological Science,* 1982, 53 (3), 557-566.

Cunningham, A. J. Information and health in the many levels of man: Toward a comprehensive theory of health and disease. *Advances,* 1986, 3 (1), 32-45.

Cupoli, J. M., Hallock, J. A., & Barness, L. A. Failure to thrive. *Current Problems in Pediatrics,* 1980, 10, (11), 1-43.

Dalton, A. J., & Selye, H. Blood picture during alarm reaction. *Folia Haematologica,* 1939, 62, 397-407.

Drugan, R. C., Maier, S. F., Skolnick, P., Paul, S. M., & Crawley, J. N. An anxiogenic benzodiazepine receptor ligand induces learned helplessness. *European Journal of Pharmacology,* 1985, 113 (3), 453-457.

Dupont, A., Barden, N., Cusan, L., Mérand, Y., Labrie, F., & Vaudry, H. Beta-endorphin and met-enkephalins: Their distribution, modulation by estrogens and haloperidol, and role in neuroendocrine control. *Federation Proceedings,* 1980, 39, (8), 2544-2550.

Epstein, G. The image in medicine: Notes of a clinician. *Advances,* 1986, 3 (1), 22-31.

Field, T., & Reite, M. Children's responses to separation from mother during the birth of another child. *Child Development,* 1984, 55 (4), 1308-1316.

Fitzgerald, M. Monoamines and descending control of nociception. *Trends in Neurosciences,* 1986, 9, (2), 51-52.

Fraioli, F., Isidori, A., & Mazzetti, M. (Eds.), *International Symposium on Opioid Peptides in the Periphery (1984: Rome). Opioid peptides in the periphery.* New York: Elsevier Science Publishers, 1984.

Gebhart, G. F. Opiate and opioid peptide effects on brain stem neurons: Relevance to nociception and anti-nociceptive mechanisms. *Pain,* 1982, 12 (2), 93-140.

Ghanta, V. K., Hiramoto, R. N., Solvason, H. B., & Spector, N. H. Neural and environmental influences on neoplasia and conditioning of NK activity. *Journal of Immunology,* 1985, 135 (2 Suppl.), 848s-852s.

Hall, H. R. Hypnosis and the immune system: A review with implications for cancer and the psychology of healing. *American Journal of Clinical Hypnosis,* 1982-1983, 25 (2-3), 92-103.

Harlow, C. M., & Selye, H. Blood picture in the alarm reaction. *Proceedings of the Society of Experimental Biology and Medicine,* 1937, 36, 141-144.

Holden, C. Cancer and the mind: How are they connected? *Science,* 1978, 200 (4348), 1363-1369.

Hung, C. Y., Lefkowitz, S. S., & Geber, W. F. Interferon inhibition by narcotic analgesics. *Proceedings of the Society for Experimental Biology and Medicine,* 1973, 142 (1), 106-111.

Jemmott, J. G., 3d, & Locke, S. E. Psychosocial factors, immunologic mediation, and human susceptibility to infectious diseases: How much do we know? *Psychological Bulletin,* 1984, 95 (1), 78-108.

Jemmott, J. B., 3d, Borysenko, J. Z., Borysenko, M., McClelland, D. C., Chapman, R., Meyer, D., & Benson, H. Academic stress, power motivation, and decrease in secretory rate of salivary secretory immunoglobulin A. *Lancet,* 1983, 1 (8339), 1400-1402.

Kalin, N. H., & Carnes, M. Biological correlates of attachment bond disruption in humans and nonhuman primates. *Progress in Neuro-Psychopharmacology and Biological Psychiatry,* 1984, 8 (3), 459-469.

Khachaturian, H., Lewis, M. E., Schäfer, M. K. H., & Watson, S. J. Anatomy of the CNS opioid systems. *Trends in Neurosciences,* 1985, 8, 111-119.

Kiecolt-Glaser, J. K., Garner, W., Speicher, C., Penn, G. M., Holliday, J., & Glaser, R. Psychosocial modifiers in immunocompetence in medical students. *Psychosomatic Medicine,* 1984a, 46 (1), 7-14.

Kiecolt-Glaser, J. K., Ricker, D., George, J., Messick., G., Speicher, C. E., Garner, W., & Glaser, R. Urinary cortisol levels, cellular immunocompetency, and loneliness in psychiatric inpatients. *Psychosomatic Medicine,* 1984b, 46 (1), 15-23.

Kobasa, S. C. Stressful life events, personality, and health: An inquiry into hardiness. *Journal of Personality and Social Psychology,* 1979, 37 (1), 1-11.

Kobasa, S. C., Maddi, S. R., & Kahn, S. Hardiness and health: A prospective study. *Journal of Personality and Social Psychology,* 1982, 42 (1), 168-177.

Kronfol, Z., Nasrallah, H. A., Chapman, S., & House, J. D. Depression, cortisol metabolism and lymphocytopenia. *Journal of Affective Disorders,* 1985, 9 (2), 169-173.

Laudenslager, M., Capitanio, J. P., Reite, M. Possible effects of early separation experiences on subsequent immune function in adult macaque monkeys. *American Journal of Psychiatry,* 1985, 142 (7), 862-864.

Laudenslager, M. L., Reite, M., & Harbeck, R. J. Suppressed immune response in infant monkeys associated with maternal separation. *Behavioral and Neural Biology,* 1982, 36 (1), 40-48.

Leshner, A. I., Merkel, D. A., & Mixon, J. F. Pituitary-adrenocortical effects on learning and memory in social situations. In J. L. Martinez, R. A. Jensen, R. B. Messing, H. Rigter, & J. L. McGaugh (Eds.), *Endogenous Peptides and Learning and Memory Processes.* New York: Academic Press, 1981, 159-179.

Levine, S. A coping model of mother-infant relationships. In S. Levine & H. Ursin (Eds), *Coping and Health.* New York: Plenum Press, 1980, 87-99.

Levy, S. The expression of affect and its biological correlates: Mediating mechanisms of behavior and disease. In C. VanDyke, L. Temoshok, & L. S. Zegans (Eds.), *Emotions in Health and Illness: Applications to Clinical Practice.* Orlando: Grune & Stratton, 1984, 1-18.

Locke, S., & Kraus, L. Modulation of natural killer cell activity by life stress and coping ability. In S. M. Levy (Ed.), *Symposium on Behavioral Biology and Cancer. National Institutes of Health, 1981. Biological Mediators of Behavior and Disease: Neoplasia.* New York: Elsevier Science Publishing Co., Inc., 1982, 3-28.

Locke, S. E., Kraus, L., Leserman, J., Hurst, M. W., Heisel, J. S., & Williams, R. M. Life change stress, psychiatric symptoms, and natural killer cell activity. *Psychosomatic Medicine,* 1984, 46 (5), 441-453.

Luk'ianenko, V. I. The problem of a conditioned reflex regulation of immunobiologic reactions. *Uspekhi Sovremennoi Biologii (Moskva),* 1961, 51, 170-187.

MacLennan, A. J., & Maier, S. F. Coping and the stress-induced potentiation of stimulant stereotypy in the rat. *Science,* 1983, 219 (4588), 1091-1093.

Maier, S. F. Learned helplessness and animal models of depression. *Progress in Neuropsychopharmacology and Biological Psychiatry,* 1984, 8 (3), 435-446.

Maier, S. F., & Seligman, M. E. P. Learned helplessness: Theory and evidence. *Journal of Experimental Psychology [General],* 1976, 105 (1), 3-46.

Maier, S. F., Drugan, R. C., Grau, J. W., Hyson, R., MacLennan, A. J., Moye, T., Madden, J., & Barchas, J. D. Learned helplessness, pain inhibition, and the endogenous opiates. In P. Harzem & M. D. Zeiler, (Eds.), *Advances in Analysis of Behavior,* Vol. 4. New York: John Wiley and Sons, 1983, 275-323.

Mason, J. W. A historical view of the stress field. (First of two parts). *Journal of Human Stress,* 1975a, 1 (1), 6-12.

Mason, J. W. A historical view of the stress field. (Second of two parts). *Journal of Human Stress,* 1975b, 1 (2), 22-36.

McClelland, D. C., Alexander, C., & Marks, E. The need for power, stress, immune function, and illness among male prisoners. *Journal of Abnormal Psychology,* 1982, 91 (1), 61-70.

McClelland, D. C., Floor, E., Davidson, R. J., & Saron, C. Stressed power motivation, sympathetic activation, immune function, and illness. *Journal of Human Stress,* 1980, 6 (2), 11-19.

McClelland, D. C., & Jemmott, J. D., 3d. Power motivation, stress and physical illness. *Journal of Human Stress,* 1980, 6 (4), 5-15.

Miczek, K. A., DeBold, J. F., & Thompson, M. L. Pharmacological, hormonal, and behavioral manipulations in the analysis of aggressive behavior. *Progress in Clinical and Biological Research,* 1984, 167, 1-26.

Miczek, K. A., & O'Donnell, J. M. Intruder-evoked aggression in isolated and nonisolated mice: Effects of psychomotor stimulants and L-dopa. *Psychopharmacology (Berlin),* 1978, 57 (1), 47-55.

Miczek, K. A., Thompson, M. L., & Shuster, L. Opioid-like analgesia in defeated mice. *Science,* 1982, 215 (4539), 1520-1522.

Miczek, K. A., Thompson, M. L., & Shuster, L. Naloxone injections into the periaqueductal grey area and arcuate nucleus block analgesia in defeated mice. *Psychopharmacology (Berlin),* 1985, 87 (1), 39-42.

Miller, N. E. Behavioral medicine: Symbiosis between laboratory and clinic. *Annual Review of Psychology,* 1983, 34, 1-31.

Mineka, S., & Henderson, R. W. Controllability and predictability in acquired motivation. *Annual Review of Psychology,* 1985, 36, 495-529.

Minor, T. R., Jackson, R. L., & Maier, S. F. Effects of task-irrelevant cues and reinforcement delay on choice-escape learning following inescapable shock: Evidence for a deficit in selective attention. *Journal of Experimental Psychology: Animal Behavior Processes,* 1984, 10 (4), 543-556.

Monjan, A. J. Stress and immunologic competence: Studies in animals. In R. Ader (Ed.), *Psychoneuroimmunology.* New York: Academic Press, 1981, 185-228.

Moretti, C., Perricone, R., De Sanctis, G., De Carolis, C., Fabbri, A., Gnessi, L., Fraioli, F., & Fontana, L. Endorphins: Evidence of multiple interactions with the immune system. In F. Fraioli, A. Isidori, & M. Mazzetti (Eds.), *International Symposium on Opioid Peptides in the Periphery (1984: Rome). Opioid Peptides in the Periphery.* New York: Elsevier Science Publishers, 1984, 137-157.

Olness, K. Imagery (self-hypnosis) as adjunct therapy in childhood cancer: Clinical experience with 25 patients. *American Journal of Pediatric Hematology/Oncology,* 1981, 3 (3), 313-321.

Overmier, J. B., & Seligman, M. E. P. Effects of inescapable shock upon subsequent escape and avoidance responding. *Journal of Comparative and Physiological Psychology,* 1967, 63 (1), 28-33.

Overmier, J. B., & Wielkiewicz, R. M. On unpredictability as a causal factor in "learned helplessness." *Learning and Motivation,* 1983, 14 (3), 324-337.

Peterson, C., & Seligman, M. E. P. Causal explanations as a risk factor for depression: Theory and evidence. *Psychological Review,* 1984, 91 (3), 347-374.

Porsolt, R. D., Anton, G., Blavet, N., & Jalfre, M. Behavioral despair in rats: A new model sensitive to antidepressant treatments. *European Journal of Pharmacology,* 1978, 47 (4), 379-391.

Reite, M. Maternal separation in infant monkeys: A model of depression. In I. Hanin & E. Usdin (Eds.), *Animal Models in Psychiatry and Neurology.* 1st edition. New York: Pergamon Press, 1977, 127-139.

Reite, M., Harbeck, R., & Hoffman, A. Altered cellular immune response following peer separation. *Life Sciences,* 1981, 29 (11), 1133-1136.

Riley, V. Psychoendocrine influences on immunocompetence and neoplasia. *Science,* 1981, 212 (4499), 1100-1109.

Rogers, M. P., Dubey, D., & Reich, P. The influence of the psyche and the brain on immunity and disease susceptibility: A critical review. *Psychosomatic Medicine,* 1979, 41 (2), 147-164.

Rothbaum, F., Weisz, J. R., & Snyder, S. S. Changing the world and changing the self: A two-process model of perceived control. *Journal of Personality and Social Psychology,* 1982, 42 (1), 5-37.

Sachar, E. J. Neuroendocrine abnormalities in depressive illness. In E. J.

Sachar (Ed.), *Topics in Psychoendocrinology.* New York: Grune & Stratton, 1975, 135-156.

Sachar, E. J., Cobb, J. C., & Shor, R. E. Plasma cortisol changes during hypnotic trance: Relation to depth of hypnosis. *Archives of General Psychiatry,* 1966, 14 (5), 482-490.

Schleifer, S. J., Keller, S. E., Camerino, M., Thornton, J. C., & Stein, M. Suppression of lymphocyte stimulation following bereavement. *Journal of the American Medical Association,* 1983, 250 (3), 374-377.

Schleifer, S. J., Keller, S. E., Meyerson, A. T., Raskin, M. J., Davis, K. L., & Stein, M. Lymphocyte function in major depressive disorder. *Archives of General Psychiatry,* 1984, 41 (5), 484-486.

Schleifer, S. J., Keller, S. E., Siris, S. G., Davis, K. L., & Stein, M. Depression and immunity. Lymphocyte function in ambulatory depressed patients, hospitalized schizophrenic patients, and patients hospitalized for herniorrhaphy. *Archives of General Psychiatry,* 1985, 42 (2), 129-133.

Seligman, M. E. P. Depression and learned helplessness. In R. J. Friedman & M. M. Katz (Eds.), *The Psychology of Depression: Contemporary Theory and Research.* Washington, D. C.: V. H. Winston & Sons, 1974, 83-113.

Seligman, M. E. P. *Helplessness: On Depression, Development, and Death.* San Francisco, California: Freeman, Cooper & Co., 1975.

Seligman, M. E. P., Weiss, J. M., Weinraub, M., & Schulman, A. Coping behavior: Learned helplessness, physiologic change and learned inactivity. *Behavioral Research and Therapy,* 1980, 18 (5), 459-512.

Selye, H. A syndrome produced by diverse nocuous agents. *Nature (London),* 1936, 138 (3479), 32. [Letter]

Selye, H. The general adaptation syndrome and the diseases of adaptation. *Journal of Clinical Endocrinology,* 1946, 6 (2), 117-230.

Shavit, Y., Depaulis, A., Martin, F.C., Terman, G.W., Pechnick, R.N., Zane, C.J., Gale, R.P., & Leibeskind, J.C. Involvement of brain opiate receptors in the immune-suppressive effect of morphine. *Proceedings of the National Academy of Sciences, U.S.A.,* 1986, 83(18), 7114-7117.

Shavit, Y., Lewis, J. W., Terman, G. W., Gale, R. P., & Liebeskind, J. C. Endogenous opioids may mediate the effects of stress on tumor growth and immune function. *Proceedings of the Western Pharmacological Society,* 1983, 26, 53-56.

Shavit, Y., Lewis, J. W., Terman, G. W., Gale, R. P., & Liebeskind, J. C. Opioid peptides mediate the suppressive effect of stress on natural killer cell cytotoxicity. *Science,* 1984, 223 (4632), 188-190.

Shavit, Y., Terman, G. W., Martin, F. C., Lewis, J. W., Liebeskind, J. C., & Gale, R. P. Stress, opioid peptides, the immune system, and cancer. *Journal of Immunology,* 1985, 135 (2 Suppl.), 834s-837s.

Sherman, A. D., Allers, G. L., Petty, F., & Henn, F. A. A neuropharmacologically-relevant animal model of depression. *Neuropharmacology,* 1979, 18 (11), 891-893.

Sherman, J. E., Strub, H., & Lewis, J. W. Morphine analgesia: Enhancement by shock-associated cues. *Behavioral Neuroscience,* 1984, 98 (2), 293-309.

Silva, A., Bonavida, B., & Targan, S. Mode of action of interferon-mediated modulation of natural killer cytotoxic activity: Recruitment of pre-NK cells and enhanced kinetics of lysis. *Journal of Immunology,* 1980, 125 (2), 479-484.

Simonton, O. C., Matthews-Simonton, S., & Creighton, J. L. *Getting Well Again.* Los Angeles, California: Tarcher, 1978.

Simonton, O. C., Matthews-Simonton, S., & Sparks, T. F. Psychological intervention in the treatment of cancer. *Psychosomatics,* 1980, 21 (3), 226-227, 231-233.

Solomon, G. F. Early experience and immunity. *Nature (London),* 1968, 220 (169), 821-822.

Stanton, M. E., Patterson, J. M., & Levine, S. Social influences on conditioned cortisol secretion in the squirrel monkey. *Psychoneuroendocrinology,* 1985, 10 (2), 125-134.

Stein, M., Keller, S., & Schleifer, S. The hypothalamus and the immune response. In H. Weiner, M. A. Hoffer, & A. J. Stunkard (Eds.), *Brain, Behavior and Bodily Disease.* New York: Raven Press, 1981, 45-65.

Stein, M., Keller, S. E., & Schleifer, S. J. Stress and immunomodulation: The role of depression and neuroendocrine function. *Journal of Immunology,* 1985, 135 (2 Suppl.), 827s-833s.

Suomi, S. J., Collins, M. L., & Harlow, H. F. Effects of permanent separation from mother on infant monkeys. *Developmental Psychology,* 1973, 9 (3), 376-384.

Suomi, S. J., Mineka, S., & LeLizio, R. D. Short- and long-term effects of repetitive mother-infant separations on social development in Rhesus monkeys. *Developmental Psychology,* 1983, 19 (5), 770-786.

Taylor, S. E. Adjustment to threatening events: A theory of cognitive adaptation. *American Psychologist,* 1983, 38 (11), 1161-1173.

Tecoma, E. S., & Huey, L. Y. Psychic distress and the immune response. *Life Sciences,* 1985, 36 (19), 1799-1812.

Terman, G. W., Shavit, Y., Lewis, J. W., Cannon, J. T., & Liebeskind, J. C. Intrinsic mechanisms of pain inhibition: Activation by stress. *Science,* 1984, 226 (4680), 1270-1277.

Visintainer, M. A., Volpicelli, J. R., & Seligman, M. E. P. Tumor rejection in rats after inescapable or escapable shock. *Science,* 1982, 216 (4544), 437-439.

Wadden, T. A., & Anderson, C. H. The clinical use of hypnosis. *Psychological Bulletin,* 1982, 91 (2), 215-243.

Watkins, L. R., & Mayer, D. J. Organization of endogenous opiate and non-opiate pain control systems. *Science,* 1982, 216 (4551), 1185-1192.

Watkins, L. R., Cobelli, D. A., & Mayer, D. J. Classical conditioning of front paw and hind paw footshock induced analgesia (FSIA): Naloxone reversibility and descending pathways. *Brain Research,* 1982, 243 (1), 119-132.

Watkins, L. R., Cobelli, D. A., Newsome, H. H., & Mayer, D. J. Footshock induced analgesia is dependent neither on pituitary nor sympathetic activation. *Brain Research,* 1982, 245 (1), 81-96.

Watkins, L. R., Drugan, R., Hyson, R. L., Moye, T. B., Ryan, S. M., Mayer, D. J., & Maier, S. F. Opiate and non-opiate analgesia induced by inescapable tail-shock: Effects of dorsolateral funiculus lesions and decerebration. *Brain Research,* 1984, 291 (2), 325-336.

Weiss, J. M., & Simson, P. G. Neurochemical basis of stress-induced depression. *Psychopharmacology Bulletin,* 1985, 21 (3), 447-457.

Weiss, J. M., Goodman, P. A., Losito, B. G., Corrigan, S., Charry, J. M., & Bailey, W. H. Behavioral depression produced by an uncontrollable stressor: Relationship to norepinephrine, dopamine, and serotonin levels in various regions of rat brain. *Brain Research Reviews,* 1981, 3, 167-205.

Glossary

Accessory cell: One of a group of immune cells, other than lymphocytes, that facilitates T cell-mediated immune reactions and antibody formation by B cells.

Acetylcholine (ACh): A major neurotransmitter in both central and peripheral (autonomic) nervous systems, acetylcholine functions in synaptic transmission in the brain and is released from parasympathetic, cholinergic nerve endings at neuromuscular junctions.

Adrenocorticotropic hormone (ACTH): Hormone secreted by the anterior pituitary gland, which stimulates glucocorticoid steroid hormone production by the adrenal cortex.

Adrenal fasciculata cell: Cells of the larger, intermediate zone of the adrenal cortex (zona fasciculata) secrete the steroid hormones, cortisol and corticosterone, as well as small quantities of sex hormones.

Adrenal gland: Endocrine gland consisting of an inner medulla and an outer cortex. The adrenal cortex secretes the glucocorticoid hormones, cortisol, corticosterone, the sex hormones (androgens and estrogens), and the mineralocorticoid, aldosterone. The adrenal medulla secretes the catecholamine neurotransmitters, epinephrine and norepinephrine.

Adrenergic pathways: Nerve tracts within the central nervous system and sympathetic branch of the autonomic nervous system, which secrete the catecholamine transmitter substances, epinephrine and norepinephrine.

Afferent nerve fiber: Ascending (centripetal) sensory nerve fiber and its processes.

Agonist: An exogenous chemical substance (e.g., drug) capable of promoting a physiologic process, such as ligand-receptor binding, or cellular secretion, in a manner comparable to its endogenous counterpart.

Allergy: Hypersensitive immune reaction to an environmental antigen.

Alloantigen: A histocompatibility antigen in transfused blood, or transplanted tissue, that is sufficiently foreign from the histocompatibility antigen complex of the host to cause rejection.

Allogenic skin graft [see Allograft]

Allograft: Tissue transplantation between different species or between individuals of the same species with different genotypes. The likelihood of aversive (allogenic) reaction and tissue rejection is minimized by a close matching of histocompatibility antigens.

Amino acid: An organic compound, composed of nitrogen, carbon, hydrogen, and oxygen. The building blocks of proteins, amino acids are bound together by peptide bonds.

Amnesia: Loss of memory. Amnesia may be complete or partial, and may be associated with epileptic seizures or other neurologic disorders.

Amygdala (amygdaloid nucleus): An almond-shaped group of nerve cells within the limbic lobe of the brain. Connected to both thalamus and hypothalamus, the amygdala, a control center for complex motor responses associated with feeding behavior, is also designated a part of the "emotional brain."

Analgesia: Diminution or absence of pain sensitivity.

Anamnestic response [see Memory, immunologic]

Anaphylaxis (immediate hypersensitivity response): A rapid, severe allergic reaction upon reexposure to antigen (allergen) following sensitization. Preformed allergen-specific antibodies, absorbed on the surface of mast cells, stimulate the release of chemical mediators (e.g., histamine) which exert powerful physiologic effects. Systemic manifestations include breathing difficulties, itching, erythema, vomiting, and diarrhea. Unless treated, symptoms can lead to bronchial and laryngeal spasm, tenesmus, and circulatory collapse.

Anastomosis: The functional union of blood vessels (i.e., capillary to capillary, arteriole to venule), or, by extension, the union of nerve fibers originating from separate nerves.

Anterior hypophysis: Anterior pituitary gland. Connected to the hypothalamus by means of a capillary plexus extending the length of the pituitary stalk, the anterior hypophysis is the source of a number of tropic hormones, which control the secretory activity of the endocrine glands.

Antibody: A protein molecule produced by plasma cells (activated B cells) that has specificity for the molecular conformation of a particular antigen.

Antibody-dependent cell-mediated cytotoxicity (ADCC): Cell lysis (cell death) brought about by mononucleated cells (K cells) towards IgG antibody-coated target cells.

Antibody-mediated immunity [see Humoral immunity]

Antibrain antibody: Autoantibody capable of crossing the blood-brain barrier and reacting against cells of the central nervous system.

Antigen: Any foreign substance that induces an immune response. Antigens include infectious agents (e.g., microorganisms), as well as noninfectious agents (e.g., synthetic polymers).

Antigenic determinant: The portion of the molecular structure of an antigen that is capable of combining with antibody. [see Epitope; Paratope]

Antiidiotypic antibody: Immunoglobulin (antibody) with determinant sites corresponding to those on the antibody molecule initially raised against antigen. Excess antibody production is controlled by idiotypic-antiidiotypic inhibitory feedback circuits within the immune system. [see Idiotype]

Antineuronal antibody: An autoantibody with specificity against neurons, or constituents thereof. Antineuronal antibodies are implicated in the pathogenesis of certain diseases affecting the central nervous system.

Antinuclear antibody: Antibody directed against constituents of the cell nucleus (e.g., DNA, RNA). Detectable by immunofluorescence, antinuclear antibodies are present in serum in some rheumatic, autoimmune diseases, such as systemic lupus erythematosus and rheumatoid arthritis.

Antiserum: Antisera, prepared from human and animal plasma, contain known antibodies, and are used in immunization. Equine antirabies serum is an animal antiserum used when administration of human rabies immunoglobulin treatment is unavailable.

Aplysia: A sea snail, equipped with large sensory and motor neurons, which has made an excellent animal model in neuropeptide research, neurophysiology, and physiological psychology.

Arcuate nucleus, periventricular nucleus: A group of nerve cell bodies, situated in the ventromedial portion of the hypothalamus, which controls reflex responses of the autonomic nervous system.

Astrocyte: A type of neuroglial, with numerous extended processes, which provides structural support and nutrients to neurons. [see Neuroglial]

Athymia: Lack of a thymus gland. Athymia in infants and laboratory animals is associated with failure to thrive, and with immune incompetence due to absence of T lymphocytes.

Atriopeptin, atrial natriuretic peptide: A peptide hormone produced by monocytes in the atrial myocardium, which plays a role in control of systemic arterial pressure by promoting fluid balance and plasma electrolyte homeostasis.

Autoantibody: Immunoglobulin that reacts against self-tissue.

Autoantigen, self-antigen: Autoantigens are molecular structures on the surface membranes of body cells that define "self," as opposed to "nonself."

Autoimmunity: An aberrant immune state in which immune processes are directed against self-antigens.

B cell (B lymphocyte): A circulating white blood cell (leukocyte) that, when activated and differentiated into the antibody-producing plasma cell, mediates humoral immunity.

Basophil: A granulocytic ameboid cell (leukocyte) containing vasoactive and anticoagulant substances.

Beta-lipotropin (β-LPH): The biologically inactive parent polypeptide molecule to the enkephalins and the endorphins, itself derived from the still larger peptide molecule, pro-opiomelanocortin (POMC).

Binding site: The area of cell surface carrying the receptor for a specific molecule (ligand).

Biotechnology: The application of new techniques in cell biology (e.g., cell fusion and the production of monospecific antibodies) to the study of normal and abnormal physiologic processes.

Blastogenesis: The formation and development of lymphocytes from lymphocyte precursor cells (lymphoblasts) that have differentiated from hematopoietic stem cells in the bone marrow.

Blood-brain barrier: A specialized capillary structure inhibiting the passage of macromolecules from the general circulation into the brain parenchyma and cerebrospinal fluid. [see Choroid plexus].

Blood group antigen: Self-antigen (phenotype) controlled by allelic genes. Blood group antigens, such as O, A, B, AB, and Rh, are found on erythrocytes.

Bone marrow: Connective tissue composed of blood plasma, fat cells, and developing blood cells, including the progenitor cells of the immune system.

Brain stem: Lowermost portion of the brain, consisting of the midbrain, pons, and medulla oblongata.

Carotid arterial circulation: The main arteries and their branching structures in the neck, which transport blood to the brain.

Catatonia: A state marked by stupor, episodes of manic excitement, emotional unresponsiveness, partial analgesia, and either rigidity or "waxy flexibility" of the musculature. Catatonia is a symptom in schizophrenia.

Catecholamine: A class of neurotransmitter substances, each having a catechol nucleus and an amine group. Catecholaminergic cell bodies and fiber systems for dopamine, epinephrine, and norepinephrine reside within precisely demarcated areas of the central nervous system. The postganglionic neurons of the sympathetic nervous system also contain catecholamines, as does the adrenal medulla.

Cell fusion: Process by which an antibody-producing cell (plasma cell) and a tumor cell (so-called "immortal" cell) are fused to create a hybrid cell line carrying characteristics of both cell types. The technique offers a means by which to produce, in large quantity, monoclonal antibodies of high specificity for experimental, diagnostic, and therapeutic purposes.

Cell-mediated immunity: An immune response involving T lymphocytes of differing types, each type carrying out specific functions, such as cytotoxicity and delayed hypersensitivity. T cells bind to antigen, proliferate in response to antigen, and play an important role in modulating the activity of B cells.

Chemotactic factor: A substance released during degranulation of mast cells, which attracts leukocytes to the site of tissue trauma or inflammation.

Chlorpromazine (CPZ): A phenothiazine derivative drug used as a tranquillizer. Chlorpromazine also acts as an immunosuppressant.

Cholecystokinin (CCK): An octapeptide neurotransmitter, with highest concentrations in the neocortex, hypothalamus, basal ganglia, and brainstem. Cholecystokinin is also found in the neurohypophysis, and in the spleen. As an intestinal hormone, CCK inhibits gastric acid secretion, and stimulates gall bladder contraction and pancreatic enzyme release.

Choroid plexus: The choroid plexi are capillary networks of a specialized type found in the lateral, third, and fourth ventricles of the brain, which act as selectively permeable barriers to the passage of solutes between brain and the cerebrospinal fluid. [see Blood-brain barrier]

Classical conditioning: Classical conditioning occurs when a neutral stimulus, temporally paired with a stimulus capable of arousing a particular response, acquires the capacity to independently elicit that same response.

Corticotropin (see adrenocorticotropic hormone, [ACTH])

Corticotropin-releasing hormone (corticoliberin [CRH]): A neurohormone, produced in the paraventricular nucleus of the hypothalamus, which regulates the release of adrenocorticotropic hormone (ACTH) from the pituitary gland, and is itself regulated by inhibitory feedback of ACTH and its hormonal products, cortisol and corticosterone.

Cortisol: A glucocorticoid hormone secreted by the adrenal cortex, cortisol regulates carbohydrate, protein, and lipid metabolism, and also acts as an anti-inflammatory agent.

Cyclic AMP (cyclic adenosine monophosphate [cAMP]): A ubiquitous nucleotide, cyclic AMP acts as a "second messenger" within the cytoplasm of the cell by mediating the effects of a first messenger (hormone, or neurotransmitter) upon the distinctive functional properties of the cell. This complex chain of events, which includes the phosphorylation of proteins by cAMP-dependent kinase enzymes, is initiated by the coupling of a first messenger molecule (ligand) with its specific receptor at the cell membrane.

Cytokine: A general term denoting biologically active substances of high specificity released by both phagocytic and nonphagocytic leukocytes. [see Monokine, Lymphokine]

Cytotoxic T cell (CTL): A type of effector T lymphocyte, the cytotoxic T cell can attack a virus-infected cell only in the appropriate histocompatibility context: i.e., against cells displaying HLA Class I antigens. [see Histocompatibility antigen]

Delayed skin hypersensitivity response: A slowly-developing (48 hour) secondary reaction to skin injection of antigen to which subject has been previously exposed. Contact dermatitis is one form of delayed skin hypersensivity.

Desmosome: A cell membrane protein, which can serve as a point of contact between cells.

DiGeorge syndrome: A condition characterized by congenital aplasia, or hypoplasia, of the thymus gland, the Di George syndrome is associated with lymphopenia, a high incidence of severe infections, tetany, and hypocalcemia.

Dopamine: A neurotransmitter involved in the mediation of emotional response and in the control of complex motor activity. Dopamine is precursor to the neurotransmitter, norepinephrine.

Dysphoria: Malaise and general feeling of disquiet.

Ectoblast: Cells of the neuroectoderm, or outermost germinal layer, of the embryo. The nervous system, the external sense organs, and the epidermal tissues are derived from the neuroectoderm.

Electroencephalogram: Measurement of brain wave activity (electrical potential) by means of electrodes applied to the scalp. Electroencephalographic patterns of brain waves not only correlate with the stages of consciousness (wakeful alertness to drowsiness), stages of sleep, and coma, but also aid in the diagnosis of neurologic disorders.

Encephalitis: Inflammation of the brain.

Endocrine system: A group of glands that release hormones into the circulation, which act in highly specific ways to alter the on-going activity of other body organs and tissues.

Endocytosis: The ingestion of extracellular material by a cell through invagination of its membrane. Phagocytosis and pinocytosis are forms of endocytosis.

Endorphin: A polypeptide derivative of the prohormone, β-lipotropin. The endorphins are synthesized in the brain, pituitary gland, immune cells, and gut. As endogenous opiates that can act both as neuromodulators and hormones, the endorphins mediate analgesia, and play a role in adaptive behavior and affective disorders.

Endothelium: Layer of epithelial cells that lines the walls of the heart, blood vessels, and lymphatics.

Enkephalin: Designation for a group of opioid peptides, the methionine [Met]- and leucine [Leu]-enkephalins. Widely distributed in the brain, enkephalins are also found in the spinal cord, spleen, and gut.

Eosinophil: A granulocytic leukocyte that releases a chemotactic factor in anaphylaxis, the eosinophil is present in tissue sites of recurrent allergic reactions, and releases enzymes that counteract the pathologic effects of other mediators of antibody-mediated hypersensitivity, e.g., histamine.

Ependymocyte: A type of neuroglial cell that, in the aggregate, forms a membranous sheath lining the ventricles of the brain and the central canal of the spinal cord. [see Neuroglia]

Epitope: An antigenic determinant of known structure.

Erythromyelopoiesis: Production of red blood cells (erythrocytes) in the bone marrow.

Experimental allergic encephalomyelitis (EAE): An autoimmune encephalitis in experimental animals, used as a model for multiple sclerosis in humans. Brain inflammation and demyelination with spinal cord involvement is caused by an induced hypersensitivity reaction to injected brain tissue.

Facteur thymique serique (FTS): (serum thymic factor [STF]) Hormone-like substance produced by the thymus gland that induces the differentiation of T lymphocytes, in vitro.

Feedback, inhibitory (negative feedback): A physiologic control mechanism whereby the level of a physiologic variable (e.g., hormone, numbers of cells) moves towards a homeostatic set point, changing in a direction opposite to that of its initial change.

Galactocerebroside (GaLC): A glycolipid substance (ganglioside) found in the tissues of the central nervous system, and containing the brain sugar, cerebrogalactose.

Gamma-interferon: A hormone-like, low molecular weight protein, elaborated by T lymphocytes, epithelial cells, and macrophages in response to infectious agents. Interferon inhibits viral replication, and also serves a number of immunoregulatory functions.

Gap junction: A cluster of protein channels that allows passage of ions and small molecules between neighboring cells.

Genetic marker: Trait linked to a single gene, which can be subjected to linkage analysis in epidemiologic research.

Genotype: One or two genes, or alleles, present at a specific chromosomal locus, which determine a particular trait, or set of traits.

Germinal center: A follicle on a lymphoid organ (spleen, lymph node) in which activated lymphocytes and macrophages proliferate.

Glycoprotein: A class of conjugated proteins complexed to carbohydrates. Serum albumin, interferon, brain gangliosides, and the antigenic determinants of memory B cells are examples of glycoproteins. Glycoproteins on the surface membranes of erythrocytes are the products of genes designating blood type.

Graft-versus-host reaction: A response to transplanted tissue in which immunocompetent T cells in the donor graft recognize the histocompatibility antigens of the recipient as foreign and initiate a hypersensitivity response.

Granulocyte: A leukocyte (white blood cell) characterized by cytoplasmic granules, which release chemical mediators in an inflammatory response. Neutrophils, basophils, and eosinophils are granulocytes.

H-2 antigen: The genetic histocompatibility antigen sequence in the mouse corresponding to the human leukocyte antigen (HLA) complex.

Haplotype: Half of a complete set of chromosomes. The haplotype is the genetic contribution of each parent to a single offspring.

Hebephrenic schizophrenia: Psychotic disorder characterized by silly behavior and mannerisms, inappropriate laughter, regression, delusions, and hypochondriasis.

Hemopoietic stem cell: The progenitor cells to a number of cell types, other than the lymphocyte, including neutrophils and monocytes, eosinophils, erythrocytes, and blood platelets.

Hippocampus: A neural structure situated in the lateral ventricle of the brain, the hippocampus is part of the limbic system (rhinencephalon).

Histamine: A powerful endogenous substance released by mast cells and associated with the immediate hypersensitivity reaction and anaphylaxis. Histamine dilates the capillaries, promotes gastric acid secretion, accelerates heart rate, and stimulates smooth muscle contraction.

Histocompatibility antigen (human leukocyte antigen [HLA]): Histocompatibility antigens are cell surface proteins, specified by closely linked genes of the major histocompatibility complex (MHC), which distinguish between the tissues of individual organisms of different species, as well as between organisms of the same species.

Histocompatibility phenotype: Tissue and organ characteristics whose genotype is determined by an individual's histocompatibility genes.

HLA-A, HLA-B, HLA-C antigens (Class I antigens): Tissue antigens, produced by the A, B, and C loci of the major histocompatibility complex (MHC), and found on the surfaces of virtually all nucleated cells, excepting erythrocytes. HLA Class I antigens are involved in the rejection of foreign tissue.

HLA-D, HLA-DR antigens (Class II antigens): Tissue antigens of the major histocompatibility complex (MHC) found on the surface membranes of cells of the reticuloendothelial system: i.e., lymphocytes, histocytes, monocytes.

Hormone: A biologic catalyst, a hormone is a chemical substance produced by a gland, or cell, which, when secreted into the bloodstream, exerts a regulatory effect on other body tissues.

"Horror autotoxicus": Term introduced by Paul Erlich (1900) to convey the notion that an organism's immunologic armament does not react against self components. The later discovery of autoimmune phenomena amended this notion.

Humoral immunity: That aspect of the immune response involving B lymphocytes. Stimulated out of resting phase by the presence of antigen, B lymphoblasts (plasma cells) produce antigen-specific antibodies, as well as long-lived memory cells.

Hybridoma: A hybrid cell created by the laboratory method of cell fusion. B cells cloned to produce monoclonal antibodies are hybridomas.

Hypophysectomy: Surgical removal of the pituitary gland.

Hypophysis (pituitary gland): A small, trilobed endocrine gland, connected to the base of the brain by a narrow stalk (infundibular stalk). Signals (neural and hormonal) received from the hypothalamus stimulate tropic hormone release from the hypophysis, which, in turn, influences the hormonal output of other endocrine organs.

Hypothalamic magnocellular nuclei: Cell bodies in the hypothalamus, which give rise to neurosecretory cells in the posterior lobe of the pituitary gland (neurohypophysis). The neurohormones, vasopressin and oxytocin, are products of these cells.

Hypothalamus: A structure in the basal diencephalon with multiple afferent and efferent connections to other brain areas. The hypothalamus regulates autonomic neural pathways, visceral reflexes (e.g., endocrine secretion, hunger and thirst, body temperature), emotional response, and instinctual behavior. Releasing hormones, produced by hypothalamic nuclei, exert indirect control over endocrine activity and govern the activity of a complex neurosecretory system.

Idiotypy: A system of membrane receptors or idiotypes. Essentially the components of a language by which the immune system regulates itself, idiotypes are linked in a complementary network of antibody interactions, i.e., antiidiotypic antibody, anti-antiidiotypic antibody, etc.

Immediate hypersensitivity response [see Anaphylaxis]

Immune-associated (Ia) histocompatibility molecule: Cell surface histocompatibility marker on immune cells, which mediates host response to foreign antigen.

Immunocompetence: The ability of the host to mount an appropriate and effective response to antigen incursion.

Immunodeficiency disease: Immune defects, either congenital or acquired, resulting in recurrent infections and failure to thrive. B and/or T cells, phagocytes, and complement proteins may either be absent, or exist in low concentrations.

Immunodiffusion: A technique for quantifying serum immunoglobulin and the formation of antigen-antibody complexes by diffusing antigen solution through agar containing a known concentration of antibody with which antigen binds, thereby producing a precipitate reaction (immunoprecipitate).

Immunoelectrophoresis: Technique by which antigen and antibody are separated by exposure to an electric field, then recombined by immunodiffusion.

Immunofluroescence: A sensitive and reliable labeling technique for identifying antigens, autoantigens, antibodies, hormones, etc., in body tissue by means of antibody conjugated to a fluorescing compound.

Immunogen [see Antigen]

Immunoglobulin: A glycoprotein made up of four polypeptide chains (two light and two heavy) linked by disulfide bonds. Produced by plasma cells (mature B cells) in response to antigenic stimulation, immunoglobulins comprise five molecular classes (IgA, IgG, IgM, IgD, IgE), each having specific antigenic, structural, and functional characteristics.

Immunoglobulin G (IgG): The most prevalent antibody in serum, and a principal antibody in the interstitial spaces of the body, IgG is the only class of antibody that can cross the placenta, thereby providing fetal immunity. IgG also promotes ingestion of antigen-antibody complexes by macrophages.

Immunoglobulin M (IgM): An immunoglobulin produced in secretory tissues, capable of antigen agglutination and lysis. IgM coating of antigen stimulates antigen ingestion by phagocytes (opsonization).

Immune homeostasis: Stable interaction, both between reactive components of the immune system itself, as well as between the immune system and other physiologic systems of the body.

Infundibular corridor: Infundibular stalk connecting the three endocrine organs, the adenohypophysis (anterior pituitary), neurohypophysis (posterior pituitary), and pars intermedia, to the base of the brain by intricate neural and vascular pathways.

Instrumental conditioning (operant conditioning): Increase or decrease in the frequency or vigor of a response (skeletal or visceral) by the reinforcement (reward or punishment) which follows the occurrence of that response.

Insulin: A large polypeptide hormone secreted by the islets of Langerhans' in the pancreas, insulin controls the rate of carbohydrate, protein, and lipid metabolism.

Interferon (IFN): A protein substance (lymphokine) released by lymphocytes, which enhances host resistance to viruses by binding to viral RNA, stimulating the proliferation of macrophages and natural killers (NK) cells, and interacting with other lymphokines to regulate various immunologic functions.

Interleukin 1 (Il-1): A polypeptide compound (monokine) derived from activated macrophages, which promotes T lymphoblast differentiation to the T helper cell subclass.

Interleukin 2 (Il-2): A mediator substance (lymphokine) released by T helper cells, which affects the proliferation and differentiation of B lymphocytes, T suppressor cells, and cytotoxic T lymphocytes (CTLs).

Juxtaglomerular apparatus: A group of cells, situated in the afferent arterioles leading to the nephron of the kidney, which secrete the proteolytic enzyme, renin.

Keratinocyte: An epidermal cell that synthesizes keratin, the principal protein constituent of skin, hair, and nails. A thymic-like hormone, produced by keratinocytes, suggests an immunologic role for these cells.

Langerhans' cell: An epidermal dendritic cell with accessory cell function. Langerhans' cells of the skin display Ia antigens and interleukin 2 receptors and participate in cutaneous cell-mediated immune reactions.

Leukocyte: A white (colorless) blood cell. Leukocytes are classified as granulocytes (i.e., neutrophils, eosinophils, basophils), and nongranulocytes (i.e., lymphocytes, monocytes).

Ligand [see Antigenic determinant, Epitope]

Limbic system (rhinencephalon): A group of interconnected neural structures, including the hippocampus, amygdala, and basal ganglia, controlling a range of autonomic, "visceral" functions, as well as voluntary movements, emotional reactions, and memory.

Linkage: The association of two or more forms of a gene (alleles), located on the same chromosome, which are inherited as a unit.

Locus: A chromosomal region, which may encompass two or more loci.

Locus coeruleus: Cell bodies in this pigmented area on the floor of the fourth ventricle of the brain synthesize the neurotransmitter, norepinephrine, and are one point of origin of a diffuse noradrenergic fiber system in the brain.

Luteinizing hormone (LH): Hormone secreted by the anterior hypophysis, which stimulates both the development of the corpus luteum in the female, and testicular cells in the male.

Luteinizing hormone-releasing hormone (LHRH): Hormone synthesized in the hypothalamus, which stimulates the secretion of the tropic hormone, luteinizing hormone (LH) from the pituitary gland.

Lymph: Transparent fluid from the interstitial spaces containing lymphocytes, macrophages, and particulate tissue debris, that, once transported through lymphatic vessels and the lymphoid organs, is delivered to the venous circulation through the thoracic ducts.

Lymph node: A lymphoid organ that occurs at intervals along the channels of lymphatic drainage. Lymph nodes filter circulating lymph, and contain germinal areas for the proliferation of lymphocytes.

Lymphatic vessels: Channels through which lymph is carried to and from the lymphoid organs, as well as to the systemic circulation.

Lymphoblast: Immature lymphocyte from which two lymphocyte lineages diverge, i.e., the T (thymus-derived) lymphocyte and the B (bone marrow-derived) lymphocyte.

Lymphocyte: Nucleated, white blood cell (leukocyte) with receptor structures (antibody, or antibody-like molecules) on its surface membrane to enable the recognition of potential pathogens.

Lymphoid organ: One of a system of organs and tissues of the immune system, including the lymphatic vessel tree, the thymus gland, spleen, lymph nodes, adenoids, tonsils, appendix, and Peyer's patches of the small intestine.

Lymphokine (cytokine): A soluble, hormone-like product of T lymphocytes. Chemotactic factor, interferon (IFN), lymphotoxin, and macrophage-activating factor (MIF) are lymphokines.

Lymphopenia: Diminished numbers of lymphocytes.

Macrophage: This large mononuclear, phagocytic cell plays an important accessory role in cell-mediated immunity by presenting partially phagocytosed antigen, in association with a histocompatibility (Ia) receptor molecule, to the T lymphocyte.

Major histocompatibility complex: A gene cluster on the short arm of chromosome 6, which encodes for transplantation antigens on the surfaces of cells.

Mast cell: Granulocytic cell localized in connective tissue, whose electron-dense granules contain powerful mediator substances (e.g., histamine, heparin, and serotonin) effective in inflammatory reactions.

Median eminence: An interstitial space, intermediate to the hypothalamus and pituitary stalk, containing a capillary network and specialized ependymocytes that facilitate the transport of biologically active materials between hypothalamus, cerebrospinal fluid, and the anterior pituitary.

Melanocyte-stimulating hormone (melanotropin [MSH]): Peptide hormone secreted by the pars intermedia of the human pituitary, which controls skin pigmentation.

Memory, immunologic: An immune characteristic demonstrated by the more rapid and robust response of an organism to an antigen to which it has been previously exposed. Immunologic memory is mediated by expanded clones of B lymphocytes known as memory cells.

Microglia [see Neuroglia]

Midbrain (mesencepahlon): An area of the brainstem containing the tegmentum, substantia nigra, inferior and superior colliculi, lying midway between the brainstem pons and the diencephalon.

Mitogen: A plant substance capable of stimulating blast transformation and proliferation, as well as lymphokine production and release, in lymphocytes.

Monoamine: Class of organic molecule containing one amine group (chemical compound formed by hydrocarbon bonds). Monoamines include the transmitter substances, serotonin, dopamine, and norepinephrine.

Monoclonal antibody: Antibody, produced by cell fusion technique, which is not only antigen-specific, but has a constant binding affinity, and can be diluted to a known concentration for therapeutic purposes. Monoclonal antisera, unlike donor antisera, can be selected to react with a high degree of specificity against particular antigenic-binding sites.

Monocyte: The large, mononuclear phagocytic cell, produced in the bone marrow, that, having once migrated to connective tissue, differentiates into the macrophage.

Monokinen (cytokine): The monokines are immunoregulatory and effector substances, as well as a group of enzymes, released by activated macrophages. Monokines include interleukin 1, prostaglandins, pyrogen, interferon, and lysozyme.

Multiple sclerosis (MS): A relapsing neurologic disease characterized by inflammatory demyelination in areas of the central nervous system, as well as alterations in the relative proportion of immunoregulatory cells. Abnormally low concentrations of T suppressor cells are a common finding in MS patients.

Myelin: A fat-like substance that is a principal constituent of the myelin sheath surrounding nerve cells. The myelin sheath promotes the conduction of nervous impulse.

Myelin basic protein (MBP): A glycoprotein found in the myelin sheath of neurons, MBP is associated with autoimmune demyelinating neuropathy.

Natural killer cell (NK cell): A cytotoxic null cell of undefined lineage, which specifically attacks cancer and virus-infected cells by contact lysis without prior sensitization.

Neocortex: The largest region of the cerebral cortex, the neocortex controls higher cortical function.

Neural crest: A band of embryonic cells that develops into the cranial and spinal nerves and adrenal medulla, the neural crest is also a site of derivation of neurosecretory cells.

Neurocytotoxic antibody: Immunoglobulin (autoantibody) that binds to neural antigens (e.g., DNA, RNA), thereby destroying neurons.

Neuroectoderm [see Ectoblast]

Neuroendocrine hormone (neurohormone): A regulatory peptide, which can behave both as a neurotransmitter (a conductor of nervous impulse), and as a hormone (whose effects upon target tissue are relatively more potent and longer-lasting).

Neuroglia: Specialized cells within the central nervous system that supply a supportive, sponge-like matrix to neurons, contributing to their metabolic requirements, and facilitating impulse transmission. Microglial cells, astrocytes, and oligodendrocytes are neuroglia.

Neurohypophysis: Posterior lobe of the pituitary gland containing a nerve bundle (hypothalamo-hypophysial tract) originating in the supraoptic and paraventricular nuclei of the hypothalamus. The neurohypophysis releases the products of these two nuclei, the neurohormones, vasopressin (antidiuretic hormone [ADH]) and oxytocin.

Neuroimmunomodulation: Effects upon the immune system arising from lesions, ablation, and electrical stimulation of the brain, most apparently from select areas of the hypothalamus.

Neuron-specific enolase: An enzyme found in gut, blood serum, brain, and cerebrospinal fluid.

Neuropeptide: Peptide hormone produced by neurons and neurosecretory cells, which demonstrates neurotransmitter-like activity. Hypothalamic releasing hormones, adenohypophysial and neurohypophysial hormones secreted by the pituitary gland, and the endogenous opioids are all neuropeptides.

Neurosecretory cell: A term used to define clusters of cells located in either the parvicellular tuberoinfundibular, paraventricular, or supraoptic nuclei of the hypothalamus, which synthesize a number of neuropeptides having "releasing" properties.

Neurotransmitter: A chemical substance released into the synaptic space between nerve cells by stimulation of a presynaptic nerve ending, which then either stimulates or inhibits the electrophysiologic activity of the postsynaptic cell.

Neutrophil: A class of phagocyte present in the early phase of an inflammatory response. Attracted to the site of inflammation by chemotactic factors (e.g., complement subcomponents), neutrophils phagocytose bacteria and cellular debris.

Newcastle disease virus (NDV): Influenza-like virus that causes respiratory, gastrointestinal, and neurologic symptoms.

Nezeldorf's syndrome: Congenital thymic dysplasia associated with impaired cell-mediated immunity, but with near-normal levels of serum immunoglobulins. The condition is characterized by severe, recurrent infections.

Norepinephrine (noradrenaline [NE]): A widely distributed neurotransmitter in the central nervous system, norepinephrine is also an agent of sympathetic nervous activity, as well as a hormone released into the general circulation from the chromaffin tissue of the adrenal medulla. Norepinephrine is important in blood pressure control, muscular coordination, defensive reactions, and in the mediation of mood.

Oligodendrocyte: Neuroglial cell important to the production and maintenance of myelin surrounding the axons of nerve cells.

Operant: An emitted response, either skeletal or visceral, which can be controlled by its consequences (contingencies of reinforcement), provided that certain response criteria of measurement (i.e., frequency, rate, intensity) are met.

Operant conditioning [see Instrumental conditioning]

Opioid peptide: Naturally-occurring (endogenous) peptide, which reacts with stereospecific opiate receptor sites in brain, spinal cord, and gut to exert opiate-like effects (e.g., analgesia). The endorphins, enkephalins, and dymorphins are opioid peptides.

Opiomelanocortin: A general term designating a class of pituitary hormones resulting from the enzymatic cleavage of the macromolecular glycoprotein, pro-opiomelanocortin (POMC).

Paratope: A binding site on antibody for an antigenic determinant (epitope).

Paraventricular nucleus (PVN): A nucleus of the hypothalamus, the PVN plays an important role in food ingestion, and contains neurons that synthesize corticotropin-releasing hormone (CRH), vasopressin, and cholecystokinin (CCK).

Parenchyma: Functional, as distinguished from supportive, tissue or stroma.

Peptide: Compound formed by reaction of amino and carboxyl groups of adjacent amino acids, which as chains linked by peptide bonds, form polypeptides, i.e., proteins.

Periaqueductal grey: Grey matter surrounding the cerebral aqueduct (aqueductus Sylvii), which connects the third and fourth ventricles of the brain. The periaqueductal grey contains efferent neurons responsible for the modulation of pain.

Peritoneum: Serous membrane lining the abdominal cavity and enclosing the visceral organs.

Phagocyte: Cell having the capacity to phagocytose (ingest) extracellular, particulate matter. Phagocytes include macrophages and polymorphonuclear leukocytes.

Phenotype: An individual's biophysical makeup, as determined by genes. Inherited characteristics, variously expressed, can reflect different phenotypes with identical genotype.

Pituitary-adrenal axis: Control axis by which endocrine hormones, stimulated into production by tropic hormones of the pituitary gland, modulate pituitary hormonal output through inhibitory feedback.

Pituitary gland [see Hypophysis]

Plasma cell: Fully differentiated, antibody-producing cell derived from the B lymphocyte.

Pleomorphic cell: Cell capable of changing shape even as it retains the same functional characteristics. The macrophage is pleomorphous.

Pluripotential hematopoietic stem cell: Self-renewing cells appearing in the yolk salk during embryogenesis, then in the fetal liver, and finally in the bone marrow. Daughter cells divide to become (1) stem cells; and (2) differentiated progenitor cells from which further differentiated cell lineages evolve: i.e., erythrocytes, lymphocytes, and monocytes.

Polymorphonuclear leukocyte: A fully developed granulocytes with a multilobed nucleus. Neutrophils are the most numerous of the poly-monuclear leukocytes.

Polypeptide: A chain of amino acids, or amino acid residues, linked by peptide bonds to form a protein.

Preoptic area: An area of the lateral hypothalamus situated between the optic chiasm and the anterior commissure.

Pro-opiomelanocortin (pro-opiocortin [POMC]): A large glycoprotein found in anterior pituitary endocrine cells, and in cell bodies in the arcuate nucleus of the hypothalamus. Enzymatic cleavage of this parent peptide yields adrenocorticotropin (ACTH), melanocyte-stimulating hormone (MSH), methionine [Met]-enkephalin, and β-lipotropin (β-LPH).

Prostaglandin: A class of potent, naturally-occurring aliphatic acid compounds, manufactured in most body tissues in exceedingly small amounts, but important to a number of physiologic processes, including bronchial dilatation, uterine contraction, vascular permeability, and urinary excretion. Prostaglandins are produced in the thymus, and are one of a group of cytokines released by neutrophils, mast cells, and activated macrophages.

Psychosomatic disease: Any disease for which the pathophysiologic mechanisms can be traced to psychological states marked by conflict, ex-aggerated emotion (e.g., aggression, fear, depression), and/or chronic arousal. Peptic ulcer, migraine headache, essential hypertension, and ulcerative colitis are among the disorders classified as psychosomatic.

Radioimmunoassay (RIA): Method for detecting presence of substance (hormone, antigen, antibody) in tissue fluids by means of radioactive isotope.

Receptor: A molecular structure, which serves as a recognition unit on the surface membrane of a cell, or within its cytoplasm. The binding of receptor and ligand (i.e., antigenic substance or molecule) effects change in cell activity.

Recognition molecule [see Antigenic determinant]

Regulatory cell: T suppressor (T_8) and T helper (T_4) cells are im-munoregulatory cells.

Renal tubule: Functional unit of the kidney from which urine is formed, and glucose, water, and electrolytes selectively reabsorbed.

Rheumatoid factor: An autoantibody with anti-immunoglobulin G and antiglobulin M specificity, which is present in the serum of most individuals with rheumatoid arthritis. Rheumatoid factor may also be found in normal relatives of patients with rheumatoid arthritis.

RNA: A polynucleotide, found in the nucleus and cytoplasm of cells, ribonucleic acid (RNA) stores and transmits genetically encoded information needed for protein synthesis.

Schwann cell: Schwann cells surround the axons of peripheral nerves to form an insulating, supportive myelin sheath.

Self-antigen [see Autoantigen]

Serotherapy (passive immunotherapy): Treatment of disease by injection of blood serum from an immunized subject.

Serotonin (5-hydroxytryptamine [5-HT]): A major neurotransmitter, serotonin is synthesized in raphe cell groupings of the midbrain, as well as in the hypothalamus. Serotonin is also liberated from blood platelets in peripheral tissues. It inhibits gastric acid secretion, stimulates smooth muscle, and plays a role in temperature regulation, sensory perception, and sleep onset.

Side-chain theory: A now-vindicated theory proposed by Paul Erlich at the turn of the century to explain the presence of antibodies in blood. According to the theory, antibodies are specific side chains on the surface membranes of immune cells, which are stimulated into synthetic activity and released into the circulation in great numbers by encounter with antigen.

Somatostatin (GH-RIF): A widely distributed peptide in the central nervous system, somatostatin acts as both a neurotransmitter and neurmodulator. Reductions in brain concentrations of somatostatin are found in such disorders as Huntington's disease and Alzheimer's disease. Somatostatin is also a pancreatic hormone that inhibits insulin and glucagon secretion by the pancreas.

Spleen: Largest of the secondary lymphoid organs and site of hematopoiesis, the spleen acts as a blood reservoir and filter, and contains germinal loci for both lymphoid and nonlymphoid cells.

***Staphylococcus* enterotoxin A:** An intestinal toxin produced by the microorganism, *Staphylococcus aureus*.

Stem cell [see Hemopoietic stem cell]

Stereochemistry: The study of the relationship between the spatial configuration of atoms and molecules in chemical compounds, and functional properties exhibited by the latter.

Stereocomplementarity: An optimum fit between ligand and receptor topographies.

Stereotyped behavior (stereotypy): Behavior marked by repetitive, meaningless movement and gesture.

Steroid: A family of hormones, i.e., the glucocorticoids, a single mineralocorticoid, and the sex hormones, which are synthesized in the adrenal cortex.

Steroidogenesis: Steroid hormone synthesis.

Substance P: A neurohormone found in the cerebral cortex and basal ganglia (striatum, substantia nigra), substance P is also an intestinal hormone, which mediates intestinal contraction.

Substantia nigra: The substantia nigra is a pigmented area of the midbrain (mesencephalon) containing the neurotransmitter, dopamine. Dopamine receptor abnormalities in the pathway of which the substantia nigra is a part (nigrostriatial pathway) are implicated in schizophrenia.

Supernatant: Term used to describe substances released by immune cells following their incubation in vitro with mitogens (plant lectin), virus, or antigen.

Systemic lupus erythematosus (SLE): A rheumatic disease with immunologic features, including an imbalance in regulatory lymphocytes, the presense of antinuclear antibodies, and immunoglobulin deposition in the glomerular basement membrane of the kidney. SLE patients can show multiple organ involvement, including brain.

T lymphocyte (T cell, thymus-derived): White blood cell (leukocyte) derived from bone marrow, but influenced in its early differentiation by passage through the thymus gland. Acting as effector cells in cell-mediated immunity, T lymphocyte subsets (T helper and T suppressor cells) regulate humoral immunity by influencing antibody production by B lymphocytes.

T cell line: A clone, or subset, of T lymphocytes, descended from a single precursor cell, hence characterized by the same genotype and a single antigenic specificity, or recognition structure.

T helper cell (T_4 cell): The regulatory functions carried out by T helper lymphocytes are essential to B cell differentiation and proliferation into antibody-producing plasma cells. A subset of T_4 cells also help induce the production of T suppresser cells (T_8) clones, which inhibit B cell maturation. T cell help is both indirect, i.e., mediated by T cell products, such as interleukin 2, and direct.

T suppressor cell (T$_8$ cell): A T lymphocyte which exerts negative control over B cell, T helper cell, and cytotoxic T cell activities.

Taraxein: A blood plasma protein fraction presumed to be involved in the pathogenesis of schizophrenia.

Thalamus: A portion of the diencephalon, composed of numerous nuclei, which integrates afferent sensory input from the body periphery, relaying visceral and somatic signals to the hypothalamus and frontal lobes.

Thoracic duct: A large lymphatic vessel, which drains lymph from lymphatic plexi throughout the body (excepting the right arm, right side of thorax, neck, and head) into the venous system.

Thymectomy: Surgical removal of the thymus gland.

Thymic aplasia: Lack of a thymus gland. The DiGeorge syndrome results from thymic aplasia.

Thymic factor: A not yet fully isolated, or characterized, hormone-like factor produced by the thymus gland. Thymosin alpha$_1$, thymosin β_4, and thymosin fraction 5 (TSN-5) are presently classified as thymic factors.

Thymic hormone: A class of polypeptide hormones produced by the epithelium of the thymus gland, which influences the differentiation of bone marrow cells into T lymphocytes, and is capable of restoring cellular immunity following thymectomy.

Thymocyte: Term used to describe a population of immature T lymphocytes, which migrates from the cortex to the medulla of the thymus gland as it matures, expressing distinctive cell surface molecules at each developmental stage.

Thymopoietin: A highly active polypeptide hormone produced in thymic epithelial cells, which induces the differentiation of prothymocytes (stem cells) into thymocytes. Thymopoietin is also implicated in autoimmune damage to acetylcholine (ACh) receptors at neuromuscular junctions in myasthenia gravis.

Thymus gland: A primary lymphoid organ, located in the thorax, which not only controls the ontogeny of T cell subsets, but also secretes a number of soluble hormones with potent regulatory effects on the entire immune system.

Thyroid gland: An endocrine gland, located in the neck, that regulates the metabolic rate of body tissues and cells, and maintains the concentration of serum protein-bound iodine. The thyroid produces the iodine-containing hormones, thyroxine and triiodothyronine.

Thyrotropin (thyroid-stimulating hormone [TSH]): Glycoprotein hormone secreted by the anterior hypophysis, which accelerates the synthesis of thyroid hormones by the thyroid gland. Thyrotropin is also synthesized by T lymphocytes.

Tolerance, immunologic: Immune unresponsiveness to self-tissue. A state of immune anergy, or functional inactivation, notable in fetal lymphocytes and in the neonate, as well as in certain immature immune cells throughout the life span.

Transduction: The transformation of energy from one to another form (e.g., electrical to chemical).

Transplantation antigen [see Histocompatibility antigen]

Trophoblast: The outer layer of the blastoderm (germinal membrane of the ovum), which supplies nutrients to the embryo through the uterine endometrium during the first days following blastocyte implantation.

Vasculitis: Inflammation and necrosis of blood vessels. Seen as either a primary, or secondary, manifestation of disease, vasculitis is usually initiated by an autoimmune mechanism, i.e., deposition of antigen-antibody complexes in blood vessel walls.

Vasoactive intestinal peptide (VIP): As a polypeptide hormone, produced by the islets of Langerhans' in the pancreas, VIP stimulates pancreatic activity, inhibits gastric acid secretion, and promotes glycogenesis. In the brain, VIP acts as a neuromodulator, exerting multiple effects on neurotransmitter systems. VIP is also found in the cortex of the thymus gland.

Vasopressin (antidiuretic hormone [ADH]): A neurohormone synthesized in the hypothalamus, and stored and released from neurosecretory cells in the posterior lobe of the pituitary gland. As a regulatory hormone, vasopressin promotes water resorption through the renal tubules, and regulates extracellular fluid osmolality and circulating blood volume. As a behaviorally-active neuropeptide, vasopressin plays an influential role in learning and memory processes.

Vena cava, inferior, superior: The venous trunk draining lower and upper extremities to empty into the right atrium of the heart.

Ventromedial nucleus: One of a group of nuclei in the medial region of the hypopthalamus. Permanent hyperphagia and obesity result from lesions in this nucleus.

White matter: Nerve fibers within, and connecting, the cerebral hemispheres of the brain are mostly white, i.e., myelinated, fibers. Thus, projection and association fibers in each hemisphere, and the corpus callosum (the commissure connecting the two hemispheres) are white matter.

Subject Index

Name Index

157